The Endemic Influence Of Evil Government: Illustrated In A View Of The Climate, Topography, And Diseases, Of The Island Of Minorca

Jonathan Messersmith Foltz

THE
ENDEMIC

INFLUENCE OF EVIL GOVERNMENT,

ILLUSTRATED IN A VIEW OF

THE CLIMATE, TOPOGRAPHY, AND DISEASES,

OF THE

Island of Minorca,

WITH

MEDICAL STATISTICS

OF

A VOYAGE OF CIRCUMNAVIGATION OF THE GLOBE,

AND

AN ACCOUNT OF OTHER SERVICE, BOTH ASHORE AND AFLOAT.

By J. M. FOLTZ, A.M., M.D.

SURGEON U. S. NAVY.

Reprinted from the New York Journal of Medicine and the Collateral Sciences.

NEW YORK:

J. & H. G. LANGLEY, 57 CHATHAM STREET.

—

1843.

R. Craighead, Printer,
112 Fulton-street.

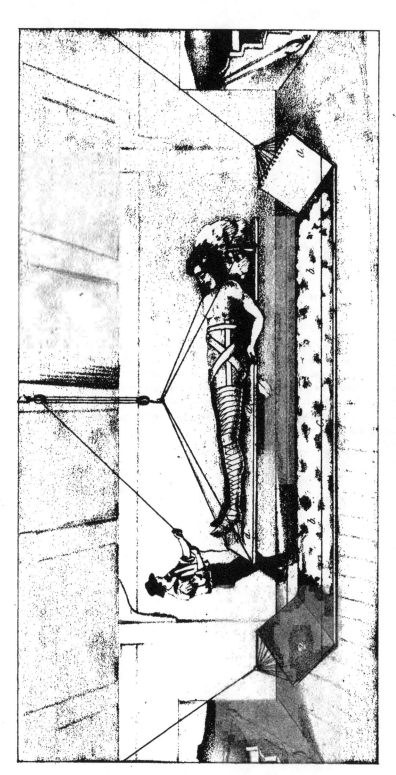

COT FOR THE TREATMENT OF FRACTURES AT SEA.

BY J.M.FOLTZ ESQ. SURGEON U.S.N.

For description see P. 45.

TO THE

HON. JAMES BUCHANAN,

OF THE SENATE OF THE UNITED STATES.

Dear Sir—

There is no one, surely, to whom I could dedicate these medical observations with more propriety than yourself; for to you I stand indebted for the kindest assistance at the commencement of my naval professional career. To you, then, I would respectfully inscribe the following pages, the result of my official duties in the most distant parts of the globe, not only as a return for kindness received, but as a feeble tribute to those distinguished talents, by which you have been enabled to fill, with such brilliant success, the many important stations to which you have been called; and trusting that still higher honors are in store for you,

I am, with great respect, your obliged friend and obedient servant,

J. M. FOLTZ,

Surgeon U. S. Navy.

ASTOR HOUSE, NEW YORK, SEPT. 1, 1843.

CONTENTS.

THE

ENDEMIC INFLUENCE

OF

EVIL GOVERNMENT,

ILLUSTRATED IN A VIEW OF

THE CLIMATE, TOPOGRAPHY, AND DISEASES OF THE ISLAND OF MINORCA,

WITH AN ACCOUNT OF

ITS MEDICAL FACULTY; OF THE FRENCH MILITARY HOSPITAL ON THE ISLE
DE LOS REYES, AND OF THE STATISTICS OF THE UNITED STATES NAVAL
HOSPITAL AT MAHON, FOR THE YEARS 1839, '40 AND '41.

THE Island of Minorca has been made familiar to the medical world by
the valuable work of Cleghorn, who held the situation of Post-Sur-
geon, at Fort St. Philip, from the year 1744 to 1749; and such is the
accuracy of his observations and the systematic regularity with which
they are recorded, that even after the lapse of a century, they constitute one of our best models for the medical observer of the present
day. At that period, the Island had for many years been one of the
most flourishing of the British Colonies, with an enterprising and pros-
perous population, numbering more than double their present amount;
while at this day, nearly half a century after its restoration to Spain,
we find poverty, wretchedness, misery, and disease, to an extent almost
incredible. In a medical point of view, these facts are of the highest
importance, affording an opportunity rarely met with, carefully to trace
the endemic influence of laws and government upon a people isolated
in consequence of being surrounded by the ocean, while the climate
and other physical causes which exercise an agency upon the human
constitution, are found to be precisely the same.

This Island having been the depot for the United States naval forces
in the Mediterranean for more than twenty years, it was found expedient to establish an hospital here, for the reception of such cases as
could not receive the necessary comforts or appropriate treatment on

board crowded ships of war. Having served as surgeon to this naval
hospital in the years 1839, '40, and '41, during which time we were
necessarily a resident of the Island, there came under our daily observation, its diseases, the character of the climate, and the condition of
the medical faculty; and as we kept a journal of events, which we
shall here endeavor to reduce to the narrowest limits, together with the
statistics of the hospital, the results cannot but be interesting to the
medical inquirer. They may moreover prove of some utility to those
who follow us upon the same grounds, or may communicate hints to
the valetudinarian who blindly rushes to the Mediterranean in search
of health, with often the sad result of thereby accelerating his death.
We humbly submit our mite towards augmenting the aggregate stock
of knowledge; and if we shall contribute but a single fact to a profession whose chief duty it is to diminish the amount of human suffering
and pain, we shall be sufficiently rewarded in the consciousness that
our labors have not been wholly in vain.

I.—THE CLIMATE, TOPOGRAPHY, AND DISEASES OF MINORCA.

Minorca is situated in 40° north latitude, and 5° east longitude from
Greenwich, and is about equidistant from the southern coasts of
Europe and the northern shore of Africa: two lines drawn, one from
Gibraltar to Rome, the other from Marseilles to Algiers, will intersect
each other at right angles on this Island. Its extreme length is thirty-
two miles, and its average breadth about fourteen, forming an irregular
oblong square, extending northwest and southeast. Its principal historical importance is due to its having been the rendezvous of Hannibal
upon his invasion of Italy. Its incomparable harbor of Mahon derives
its name from his brother Mago, who here organized a regiment of
slingers, who distinguished themselves in the Punic wars; and, for this
dexterity in the use of the sling, the peasantry are still remarkable after
a lapse of two thousand years.

In recent times, this Island has alternately belonged to Spain, France,
and Great Britain. From its peculiar geographical position and secure
port, it will likely continue to remain as a bone of contention among
the rival powers of Europe; and to France, in particular, it has become
of peculiar value, since their occupation of Algiers. The British
forces took possession of the Island in 1708, and it remained under
their power, with an interval of sixteen years, until 1802, when it was
restored to Spain in conformity to the Treaty of Amiens, having since
remained in the Spanish possession; and from that period to the present
time, it has continued to share the reverses and misfortunes of its
ill-fated parent country. We see on every side the evidence of its
former wealth and commercial prosperity,—large store-houses, extensive public buildings, good roads, and an almost impregnable fortifica-
tion, all in a state of ruin and dilapidation.

The physical characters of the Island are peculiar, and exert a strong
influence upon its vegetable and animal productions. The entire
Island is composed of calcareous limestone, presenting a bold and
rock-bound coast to the sea, with a rough and broken surface, throughout its whole extent. Its northern portion may even be said to be
mountainous; its most elevated peak, Mount Toro, having an altitude
of two thousand one hundred feet above the level of the sea.

The northern shore of the Island is indented by numerous deep bays, occasioned by the violence of the sea, whose waves, beating upon it age after age, have been urged on by the storms, which have ever been proverbial for their severity in the Gulf of Lyons; while the southern shores of the Island, which are not exposed to so heavy a surf, but are fanned by the genial airs from the coast of Africa, are regular and unbroken from end to end. A broken and hilly aspect, with naked rocks and fragments of stone, is presented over the entire surface of the Island; and its scanty soil has been carefully turned to the best account, by a diligent cultivation of their small fields, enclosed with high stone-walls. There are no streams of fresh water in the Island deserving of the name; and as the few rivulets, which during the winter season are swollen, disappear entirely during the long drought of the summer, the inhabitants are obliged to obtain water from wells for the purpose of irrigating their gardens, or to depend upon the rain water collected in the cisterns, which last is the only drinking water that they have. Each house is furnished with a cistern, in which large quantities of water are collected during the rainy season; and notwithstanding it is often kept four and six months, it is found much better than the water kept in the same manner that we have met with in other countries. Water, however, is little used by any class of the natives, as the light wines are of such abundance that all classes make them their chief drink. Coffee is so expensive as to be within the reach only of the few, and tea is never used but as a medicine. The road constructed by the English from Cendadella, on the western extremity of the Island, to Fort St. Philip on the east, divides it into nearly two equal parts, and forms the boundary between two sections of the Island, each of which is important in its medical, as well as in its physical features.

The country north of this road is rough, rocky, sterile, and unhealthy; while that to the south is more regular in its formation, more fertile, and much more salubrious. In the south are to be found many beautiful valleys, cultivated with great care, and yielding large crops of corn and wine; but there is one feature which gives to the landscape an unpleasant aspect, its destitution of trees,—a result which is attributed to the violence of the winter winds. The fig and vine, which are carefully cultivated wherever the ground is sheltered, yield their delicious fruits in abundance.

The great diversity in the fertility of the soil and in the state of agriculture, in the northern and southern sections of the country, is peculiarly exhibited in the domestic animals. Those from the south are large, well-formed, and in good condition; while those from the northern rocky shores, are stunted and poor. A mere glance at the cattle in the market renders it unnecessary to inquire from which section they came.

The mean annual temperature of Mahon is found to be higher than that of Naples or Gibraltar, in the same latitude, and washed by the same sea. This is doubtless due to the circumstances that Mahon is surrounded by the ocean, and is not, like the two former localities, exposed to the cold winds sweeping from the snow-clad mountains of Italy and of Spain. The mistral, which descends with such intense severity from the maritime Alps upon the plains below, have, on reaching Minorca, been tempered in their long passage over the sea; and although snow falls annually on the shores of the Mediterranean, yet we never saw it at Mahon. Storms of hail, however, are very frequent and very violent. It is the prevailing impression that the climate of Europe has become very much meliorated in modern days, and that the winters are neither so cold nor so protracted in duration, as during the time of the Romans. Although, in the absence of regular thermometrical observations, (the thermometer being an instrument of modern invention), we are unable, as regards the general question, to come to any precise conclusion; yet daily observations, carefully recorded at Mahon for more than a century, conclusively prove that here at least, for a period of one hundred years, the climate remains precisely the same.* Upon a careful comparison of the mean temperature of the four seasons, on an average of four years, embracing 1740 and 1840, the ratios were found to be almost precisely the same; and the record of the winds, as kept by Cleghorn, corresponds in each season of the year with those kept at the time of our residence upon the Island.

Meteorological observations are carefully made by the monks at their monasteries; and the writer would take this opportunity thankfully to acknowledge the cheerfulness with which they allowed him access to these records. A rain-gauge was not kept; but we are enabled, not-

---

* In the two works recently published by Dr. Samuel Forry, entitled " *Meteorology*," and "*The Climate of the United States and its Endemic Influences*," this question is very fully investigated. He shows, from abundant historical evidence, that ever since the time of the first Roman emperors, the climate of Europe, as regards the mean annual temperature, has experienced no appreciable change, and that the most remarkable extremes of heat and cold have been frequently recurring; and from this extensive survey of historical facts, he arrives, contrary to general opinion, at the following conclusions:

" All observations then, thus far, confirm the belief in the general stability of climates. As regards the seasons, it will be shown, however, that in countries covered with dense forests, the winters are longer and more uniform than in dry, cultivated regions, and that in summer, the mean temperature of the latter is higher. Hence, *in regard to the opinion generally entertained, that the climate of Europe has been very much meliorated since the days of Julius Cæsar, it is clearly apparent, from the foregoing facts, that it is far from being sustained by evidence sufficient to enforce conviction.* But, at the same time, while it is obvious that no material change has taken place, for the last two thousand years, in the climate of Europe, the conjecture that it has gradually acquired rather a milder character, or at least that its excessive severity seems on the whole to occur less frequently, appears to be warranted. . . . Dense forests and all growing vegetables, doubtless, tend considerably to diminish the temperature of summer, by affording evaporation from the surface of their leaves, and preventing the calorific rays from reaching the ground. It is a fact equally well known, that snow lies longer in forests than on plains, because, in the former locality, it is less exposed to the action of the sun; and hence the winters, in former years, may have been longer and more uniform. As the clearing away of the forest causes the waters to evaporate and the soil to become dry, some increase in the mean summer temperature necessarily follows."

In a work by the late Noah Webster, LL.D., still more recently published, entitled "*A Collection of Papers on Political, Literary, and Moral Subjects*," this same question is most learnedly discussed in a dissertation of forty-four octavo pages, "*On the supposed Change in the Temperature of Winter*." So general is the opinion that the temperature of the winter season, in northern latitudes, has suffered a material change, and become warmer in modern than it was in ancient times, that "*I know not*," says Dr. Webster, " *whether any person, in this age, has ever questioned the fact.*" From a most extensive examination of ancient writings, in the Hebrew, Greek, and Latin, he confirms and establishes most conclusively the deduction arrived at by Dr. Forry.

withstanding, to state the mean for the years 1839 and '40, which is forty-nine inches. The mean temperature of the year is 61°.31, and of the seasons as follows:

Spring.	Summer.	Autumn.	Winter.
58°.08	72°.80	64°.14	50°.22

The mean annual temperature is nearly two degrees higher than that of Rome, the difference being caused by a milder winter.

The winds at Minorca constitute the most important climatic feature. During the winter there is almost a continued tornado from the northwest, while in the summer months there is an almost uninterrupted calm, or light airs from the south. The sea-breeze, which sets in about eleven o'clock, A. M., is not so strong, nor so regular, as in larger islands; and inasmuch as the dwellings have all been erected with a view to protection from the northwesters, the inhabitants enjoy but little of the refreshing air from the sea, during the intensely hot and long summers. The prevailing winds are from the north and west; and violent gales come from that quarter only, carrying with them the spray of the sea, and leaving a deposit of salt upon every part of the Island. Even plants newly grown on the most elevated parts of the country, will, upon tasting them, discover this spray. The gales of the winter, which blow with terrific violence, injuring trees, walls, and houses, have for ages been the terror of the navigator; but they are generally of but a few hours' duration; and such is their effect upon the clumps of bushes and stunted trees, that their trunks and branches are always inclined to the south. The south wind is mild and gentle, and the sirocco, which is felt with great severity at the neighboring Islands of Sicily and Sardinia, never reaches here; and thus do the inhabitants possess an exemption from one of the greatest evils of the Mediterranean.

Diseases of Minorca.—The history of the diseases of Minorca, as given by Cleghorn, exhibits, as compared with the present, a complete revolution in their character within the century; and, as the same meteorological observations prove that the climate remains the same, we must look to other causes for this change in the condition of the people. These causes have obviously their origin in the *endemic* agency of bad government, and perhaps nowhere can its influence upon the moral, intellectual, and physical condition of man be so strongly and so clearly traced, as in this little Island. The laws of an inscrutable Providence seem to ordain that all nations shall carry with them the principles of youth, maturity, and decay; but in this people, the transition has been so rapid, that we may safely attribute the change, more to the oppression and tyranny of man, than to the operation of natural causes. In the change of government from freedom to oppression, accompanied with a change from activity to idleness, and from the cheerfulness of prosperity to the gloom and despondency of poverty,—we may clearly trace the cause of increased disease, infirmity, and decrepitude; and such has been the extraordinary change produced in this people within a century, that, were it not for the incontrovertible testimony of the excellent man whose work is before us, we would not be willing to give credence to what we must be convinced is the fact.

The Island at that time contained a population of forty thousand; and such was the vigor and general health of the community, that in a five years' residence, Cleghorn did not " meet with a single individual who was lame or deformed," and " cases of paralysis were of extremely rare occurrence." At present, the population is only eighteen thousand, and the streets and highways are crowded with the maimed, the halt, and the blind. The number of poor and mendicants is so great, that the inhabitants are unable to maintain an hospital. Besides, the onerous contributions and heavy taxes, levied for the support of the troops during the protracted civil war, have almost made paupers of the whole community.

A few families who still have it in their power, distribute alms on fixed days in the week, which collects all the beggars in the vicinity; and, on these occasions, we have counted upwards of one hundred and fifty from our window,—a host which must have belonged to the town alone, which contains a population of only seven thousand. Many of these beggars formerly had houses of their own; but having long been without employment, they are now without food, and are reduced by disease to the lowest stage of distress and degradation. Such of the citizens who were formerly in affluence, are at present barely able to live, and those who enjoyed the necessaries and comforts of life, are reduced to poverty. It is seldom that we have entered a dwelling, from the noblesse to the pauper, that we did not hear lamentations on account of their changed condition,—dwelling with pride upon their former wealth, and sighing over their present depressed state, from which no effort of the most industrious and frugal life can extricate them. The laws paralyze every effort of industry, the very appearance of success and thrift, even in the laborer and tradesman, being followed by increased levies from their insatiable rulers; and such callings in life, which elsewhere are disreputable and degrading, are here openly pursued by the most respectable of the inhabitants. It is no disgrace, for instance, to be engaged in smuggling, gambling, and the slave trade, the propriety of these occupations being never brought in question; and at the last of these pursuits, some large fortunes have recently been made.

The most industrious of the population have abandoned the Island, and many are still leaving, the tide of emigration flowing towards New Orleans and Algiers; and, should it continue at the same ratio in which it has gone on for several years, this Island, so much favored in its climate and harbor, will soon be literally depopulated. Two thousand persons emigrated during the year 1840; and when it is remembered that they are the young, the active, and the enterprising, leaving behind the aged, the infirm, and the helpless, its effect upon this small population must be evident. We were informed by those best capable of forming a correct judgment, that two-thirds of the community are females,—a conclusion which our own observations would confirm.

The continued operation of the depressing passions, and the want of the necessaries of life, are the causes of the vast amount of disease to be found in the present day among the inhabitants; and it is to the agency of these endemic causes that the premature old age, which obtains among these people, who at forty-five and fifty present all the decrepitude and infirmities which, on the continent, are only met with twenty years later in life, are to be ascribed. The Church itself has, doubtless, exerted an unfavorable influence upon the prosperity of the Island; for there are a large number of priests, who must necessarily be supported by those who labor; and, besides, the great number of religious festivals and holidays which are scrupulously kept, take from the natives much time, which, in their present condition, had better be devoted to some more immediately useful employment. The depreciation in the value of property is the strongest evidence of the change in the condition of the people : buildings which were formerly worth £10,000, can at present be purchased for £500; and large and comfortable dwellings may be rented for £5 per month.

Fevers.—The diseases formerly of most frequent occurrence were *fevers*, which then assumed a type never to be met with in the present day. Then they were violent in accession, rapid in their progress to malignancy, and often proving fatal within fourteen and twenty days. At present, notwithstanding fevers are common, they are almost invariably of a mild tertian form, and are only to be dreaded in their sequelæ, inasmuch as they rarely or never prove fatal of themselves.

Intermittent Fever.—This is the only form of febrile affection that came under our observation, and in four-fifths of these cases we found that they assumed the tertian type, differing materially from the intermittents of the United States. The paroxysm generally continues from ten to twelve hours, being preceded by a very short cold stage, rarely amounting to more than a slight chill or coldness of the extremities. The violent shivering common with us, is here unknown. The pyrexia is, however, much more violent : it is, in a majority of cases, accompanied with delirium, and it is invariably followed by a violent sweating stage, which prostrates the patient, and occasions great emaciation, with a deep yellow or brown complexion. From this condition, the sufferer is a long time in recovering; and when in the state of convalescence, he is peculiarly susceptible to organic disease upon slight exposure. It is these secondary affections, for which the intermittents prepare the patient, that usually prove fatal. These intermittents attack all classes, such as reside in the most comfortable dwellings in the city being no less subject to the disease than those who dwell in crowded and exposed hovels. The town, however, is more exempt from them than the country; and the farmer and laborer in the open fields, who, with their families, in most parts of the world, are blessed with more than the average proportion of health, as the inestimable prerogative of rural life, have here entailed upon them additional misery and misfortune. During the summer and autumn, when these fevers prevail, the peasantry are found in the fields with their heads bound up, feeble and exhausted, endeavoring to perform, during the remission of the paroxysm, a portion of the indispensable agricultural labor. These cases were found perfectly tractable when judiciously treated, and with prudence their return was readily prevented; but from the continued operation of the endemic causes heretofore enumerated, relapses were very frequent; and as these moral and physical agents were beyond the reach of professional advice, cases were daily presented in which the young and promising were gradually sinking under these renewed and oft-repeated attacks. Indeed, we were more frequently consulted by individuals who anticipated an attack, as to the best means of prevention, than for medicines to arrest the disease after it had once set in. The anticipations

2

of an attack, in truth, appeared much more dreadful than the actual sufferings induced by the disease after it had been once developed.

In this state of anticipated evil, the natives are in the habit of resorting to many means for the purpose of warding off the disease. Among these, charms and amulets, and also protections and immunities from the priests, hold a conspicuous rank ; and it were well if all their efforts at prevention were equally harmless. Not satisfied with these, however, they frequently drench themselves with the most powerful and drastic medicines, among which the pills of Morrison and the purgative mixture of Le Roy are in the most repute; and the amount of suffering they thus induce is incalculable, as they often develope more active and serious disease, which proves fatal, or at best procrastinates the recovery. The solution of arsenic, sold as a secret nostrum, is much used, and its fatal effects, particularly in developing dropsy, were frequently witnessed ; but of these remedies we shall have more to say, when we come to speak of the condition of the medical faculty. Simply confining the patient to his bed, and giving a few doses of the sulphate of quinine, would never fail to arrest the paroxysms. If these cases, however, were attended with much hepatic derangement, the assistance of some mild mercurial purgatives or emetic, which we have always preferred, would generally suffice to make the disease yield ; and the patient, in a few days, would be enabled to resume his ordinary avocations. It was, however, from the great liability to a recurrence, that we experienced difficulty in its management; and here we were so fortunate as to introduce a remedy, which speedily acquired great popularity, and came into general use throughout the Island.

Some years ago, while at Batavia, in the island of Java, we were informed by Dr. Fritz, for many years the surgeon of the Dutch Military Hospital there,—a locality characterized by a malignant and obstinate form of endemic intermittent,—that he found the following prescription more effectual than all others used by him; and to his warm recommendation of its use, we can add, from some experience with it in the intermittents which prevail upon the banks of our own Chesapeake as well as in Minorca, that we have found it more efficacious than quinine or any of the other preparations in ordinary use :

℞.——Pulv. Corticis Cinchonæ   .   ℥j
          Supertart. Potassæ .   .   ℥ij
          Pulv. Caryophili   .   .   ℥j
          Vini Rub: (Port)   .   .   Oj

M. Dose—One ounce to be taken every hour for six hours preceding the expected paroxysm.

This prescription was carefully preserved by the heads of most families, and was prepared by the apothecaries of the Island ; and we had the satisfaction of knowing that its simple introduction relieved many, and accomplished no little good ; but whatever degree of celebrity and reputation fell to our share in consequence, was more than counterbalanced by our horrid practice of insisting upon cleanliness, and obliging the patient to wash and shave himself,—measures which the native practitioners and patients consider very improper in this disease ; and so loyally do they act up to this belief, that an individual suffering from the tertiana in Minorca, may often be known by a long beard and an unwashed face.

Neuroses.—Next in the order of frequency, but first in point of fatality, stands that long catalogue of distressing diseases of the nervous system, termed *neuroses;* and they are to be found here, from the most insidious forms of neuralgia to the aggravated modifications of paralysis and mania. This class of affections, which, in the days of Cleghorn, were seldom encountered, are at this period the prevailing complaints. Extensive observations carefully conducted, among the residents of the interior, as well as the citizens of the town, prove that at present this class of diseases, particularly the more aggravated forms affecting the encephalon and spinal marrow, are more frequent and more fatal in their progress and termination than any other; and these affections assume every protean form, from apoplexy and mania to the milder forms of partial derangement and hypochondriasis. The number of cases of hemiplegia and paraplegia to be found in this community, far exceeds in amount the average number of any other district with which we are familiar; and they embrace every age, class, and station of society. The milder forms of monomania and mental despondency are so frequent, that the physician must be prepared to meet them in almost every adult that he is called to see; and he will find his patient anxious to detail to him his misfortunes, loss of property, pecuniary embarrassments, and the dread of approaching poverty and want; and these causes combined not unfrequently drive the poor unfortunate to suicide. In these cases, professional services are often of only temporary benefit, as the infirmities, induced by the mental distress and dejection, notwithstanding relieved for the time, will be sure to return with increased severity, as the causes still continue to operate. It is thus sufficiently obvious that here is presented a wide field for the philanthropist, who could realize even more than his brightest hopes, simply by removing the endemic agency of a bad government in the establishment of a good one.

Insanity.—In the various cases of this disease which came under our observation, a majority were found in the better classes of society. We were forcibly struck with the mild and pacific character of the patients, and we could not learn that they ever evinced symptoms of raving or furiousness in their delirium. But notwithstanding the great number of cases of mental derangement, and the milder forms of monomania, but one case of idiocy, during all our residence, was brought to our notice; and that was in a lad of sixteen, whose peculiar craniological formation strongly confirmed the suspicion of congenital cerebral defect.

A detail of these cases is forbidden by the limits of this article,—a circumstance that we much regret, as some of them, we doubt not, would prove no less interesting to the profession than they were to us; and it is with pleasure that we are enabled to record our testimony in favor of the excellent and the efficient moral treatment, which we found, in many instances, bestowed by the relatives and friends; and this, in some cases, had been continued for years upon the unfortunate sufferers. Were any additional testimony necessary to confirm the superiority and the success of the moral treatment over all others, in every stage of mental derangement, we have many cases at hand which would incontrovertibly establish the point. We shall, however, here make the acknowledgment, that in the various cases in which our advice was given, we were often compelled to attribute the restoration of the patient much more to the kind and soothing attentions of the relatives and friends, than to our remediate measures; and this, too, not unfrequently, in cases in which active and energetic measures had been rigidly enforced, such as venesection, local bleeding by cups and leeches, counter-irritants, the shower-bath, emetics, purgatives, and even a mercurial course. In almost every case that occurred in adults, the cause of the malady was pecuniary embarrassments and the fear of poverty; for, among the Spaniards of the better class, who hold that manual labor is disreputable, the state of poverty is regarded with horror; and to this unfortunate mental condition, their natural irritability of temperament and strong passions materially contributed. In two cases, the disease was brought on by disappointed love; and this, with them, is truly their ruling passion. Just before our arrival a melancholy case occurred, in which both parties were under twenty years of age. The young man, rejected by the object of his attachment, stabbed her to the heart in her father's house, in the most central part of Mahon; and it is in the operation of this passion, that the temperament of the Spaniard is found to differ so much from the cooler and more rational resident of the countries of the north, thus making him in prosperity more joyous and cheerful, in adversity more sad and dejected.

Paralysis.—As regards this disease, we believe that there were but few cases on the Island in which we were not consulted; and notwithstanding the duration and hopeless nature of the disease, we were induced to obey by the urgent, and often imploring, solicitation of the sufferers, who, bedridden or crippled for years, eagerly sought relief; being willing to submit with delight to any course of treatment which we would recommend. Persevering with different modes of treatment, we had the gratification, in several cases, of at least relieving some of the most distressing symptoms; but, in most cases, our efforts were of but little avail. To Mr. Turnbull's remedy, strychnine, we gave a most faithful trial, using it in every form both externally and internally. In many cases, the mobility of the paralyzed member was much increased, and strong muscular contractions were brought on in members which had long been immovable; but in no one case was there any permanent benefit derived from its use. The means which we found of most service, were counter-irritants, (particularly where the discharge had been kept up for some time,) and a careful attention to the general health, relieving such symptoms as from time to time required our care, and leaving the case to time and nature. The preparations of iodine, particularly the hydriodas potassæ in small doses, were at times of service. In one case of a young woman, it was of much benefit. In another case of hemiplegia, acupuncturation of the tongue was followed by a most decided improvement in the powers of articulation; nor was this change only temporary, as is so frequently the case after this operation, but the ability to articulate continued from the period of the operation until the time of our departure from the Island.

Intemperance.—This most fruitful source of disease in the United States does not here exert its baneful influence; for, however much the Minorcan may be depressed by poverty, or degraded by want of education, from this vice he at least is free; and although wine of a good quality forms the ordinary drink of all, yet it is very seldom that an individual, even of the lowest classes, is found intoxicated. This, therefore, cannot be urged as one of the causes of the frequency of paralysis among these people.

Neuralgia Facialis.—Many persons, particularly females, suffer from this affection, which often assumes an intermittent character, returning at regular periods. We have even seen it assume a tertian type; and in confirmation of its being dependent upon the same causes which produce the tertian fevers, it may be added that the treatment with quinine, piperine, and tonics, was the most effectual. Indeed, a few large doses of quinine would generally allay the most intense neuralgic pain.

Cancerous Affections.—Cancers, including *lupus,* both in males and females, as well as *caries* and *necrosis,* are of very frequent occurrence; but they are almost exclusively confined to the poorer classes, who are badly sheltered and often suffer from the want of proper food. The country residents, who are more exposed to atmospheric vicissitudes than such as live in the town, are also very liable to these affections. We find that we have memoranda of seven cases of cancer accompanied with ulceration, in three of which the disease was situated in the lip; and we met with probably as many more, which were rapidly progressing to suppuration. In one of these, a male, aged thirty-two, the disease being situated on the lip, an operation had been performed for its removal about ten months prior to our seeing the case: the cicatrix had become indurated, and presented the peculiar metallic, scaly lustre, which precedes the ulcerative stage. This patient we placed upon the use of the liquor arsenicalis of Fowler, and gradually increased the dose, until strong symptoms of the poisonous operation of the metal were manifested; and so long as the system was under the influence of the medicine, the darting pains in the lip, which were at times very severe, entirely disappeared. The unfortunate sufferer became sanguine in the hope of a restoration to health,—feelings which we carefully cherished and endeavored to strengthen. These moments of hope and cheerfulness, however, were but of short duration; for, as soon as the impression of the arsenic abated, the disease returned with increased violence, and it has, doubtless, long ere this time, proved fatal.

Lupus.—Two cases of this disease, comparatively a rare affection in other countries, and almost unknown in the United States, were here peculiarly malignant; and in this small population they far exceeded, in severity and their dreadful consequences, the most frightful ravages of the disease exhibited in the large hospitals of London and Paris. In one case, nearly all the bones of the face were involved in these fungous ulcerations; and in the other, one eye was forced from its socket, the ulceration having entirely destroyed the nose and much of the contents of one orbit. Both these patients were males, who resided in the interior of the Island, and neither had ever suffered from any specific constitutional disease, which is so frequently the forerunner of these unfortunate cases. Simple cases of lupous tubercles, accompanied by discoloration and deformity, were very common, which, as they were not attended with pain, were the only inconvenience accompanying them. Our treatment of these cases was nearly uniform, directing the ordinary alteratives, particularly the preparations of iodine; and in the cases attended with ulceration, we had the satisfaction of seeing these remedies, when combined with stimulating dressings to the ulcer, of manifest benefit; but in such cases as were unattended with ulceration, and where the tubercles were indolent, we could not observe the slightest change for the better, after the most prolonged and careful attention. In several, the disease continued to advance with steady steps, at the same time that active remedies were regularly administered. The decoction of sarsaparilla, nitric acid, the iodides of iron and potassa, with local and general baths, were each in turn ordered; and, as before stated, where ulceration had taken place, they were used with decided benefit. As a local application, after having used the various mild and soothing remedies, several of the most extensive ulcers rapidly healed under the dressings of an ointment, consisting of iodide of sulphur, grs. xv., and lard, ℥ss. These cases were most frequent in persons still in their minority, or in the prime of life; and in those individuals advanced in years, who had suffered from the disease, it appeared to have worn itself out, leaving behind the melancholy marks of its visitation. It was chiefly, however, among the poor that these cases occurred. A cast was taken in a case in which the tumor was very large, and occasioned much deformity; and by the use of this, a regular and equable pressure was maintained upon it, thus diminishing the induration very materially. It promised at first a favorable termination; but the patient did not give it that careful attention which the nature of the treatment required.

Aneurism.—This is a very common disease; and as its nature and treatment are here but little understood, it generally proves fatal. As we attribute this affection to a diseased nutrition, we may be prepared to meet many cases of it at Mahon. Those of the large arteries, near the heart, are most frequent, and seldom are they confined to a single tumor; they are rapid in their progress, and speedily prove fatal. We made a post-mortem examination, in which five large aneurismal tumors were found upon the aorta and the subclavian arteries; and in this case, the only treatment that had been pursued was Morrison's pills, and at intervals large doses of quinine.

Our introduction to our medical *confrères* of Mahon, and into practice among the natives, was owing to a case of aneurism. Very soon after our arrival, we were invited by Dr. Regal to be present at an operation for securing the femoral artery in a case of popliteal aneurism; and as this operation had not been attempted here for years, most of the faculty had assembled on the occasion. Our first impressions, we must acknowledge, left but little desire to cultivate a further acquaintance. There are, however, among them several gentlemen of liberal education, and well qualified to take a higher stand than they are destined to hold in this community. The patient, a Spanish sailor, æt. thirty, had a large aneurismal tumor in the left popliteal region, with strong pulsations in every part of it; the size of the tumor was so great, that the limb from the knee down was œdematous, and pulsations could not be perceived in the arteries below the tumor; the individual was much emaciated, and in an unfavorable condition to undergo the operation. In dividing the superficial layers, much time was unnecessarily consumed, and unfortunately, the vein was opened, which produced a profuse hæmorrhage. After much delay, sponging, and tearing, the surgeon was unable to secure the artery. At this stage of the proceedings, our assistance was requested; and from the unfavorable condition of the case, we recommended immediate amputation. This, however, would not for a moment be listened to, either by the medical attendants or the patient. We, therefore, proceeded to make a fresh incision two inches higher, and passed a ligature around the artery, which, as soon as secured, arrested the hæmorrhage and pulsations in the tumor. The patient was now placed in bed, directed to be kept quiet, and one drachm of infusion of digitalis ordered every four hours. Notwithstanding the unfavorable prognosis, the case continued to do well until the twelfth day, when violent pain set in, which terminated in mortification of the foot. The ligature came away on the eighteenth day after the operation, and soon after, the line of demarcation distinctly formed in the middle of the leg; and, after months of suffering, the mortified parts were completely detached, leaving a very clever stump.

The unpleasant duty here devolves upon us to record the death of one of the most affluent and useful citizens of Mahon, in consequence of the officious interference of an ignorant surgeon, in a case of popliteal aneurism. M. Vidal, aged fifty, had enjoyed uninterrupted health for many years, devoting his time to the management of his estates and the enjoyment of domestic comforts. Discovering a small tumor under the knee, which gave him no uneasiness as it was unaccompanied by pain, he, nevertheless, as it continued to increase, sent for his medical attendant, who pronounced it an imposthume, declaring that he distinctly felt the fluctuation within. Promising to call again and open it, which he assured his too credulous patient would at once relieve him, he accordingly did so in the evening; and boldly plunging a lancet into the supposed imposthume, he opened the cavity of an aneurismal sac which was, of course, immediately followed by a copious hæmorrhage. By means of compress and bandage, he succeeded in arresting the bleeding for a time; and now leaving the patient in bed, he assured him that all was just as he had anticipated. The exhausted patient soon fell into a profound sleep, the hæmorrhage recurred, and during the night he awoke and found himself weltering in his blood. Scarcely able to articulate, time was only allowed to administer the last rites of the Roman church when the unfortunate patient expired.

In several cases of aneurism, in which we were consulted, we had the gratification by a rigid perseverance in the antiphlogistic regimen, venesection, perfect rest, and digitalis, as recommended by Valsalva, of seeing the most happy results follow. In the case of a watchmaker, the individual was enabled, after some time, to resume his usual avocations, and contribute to the support of his family.

Aneurism by Anastomosis.—A few cases of congenital aneurism came under our care; but they are not more frequent here than elsewhere. In their removal we rarely had recourse to the knife, as we found the natives invariably recovered slowly from operations; and, as regards union by the first intention, we do not remember having ever witnessed it, however small the lesion may have been. When these cases of nævi materni occurred in children, little difficulty was experienced in destroying them by repeated applications of the caustic potassa. We always took especial care to insert it well within the enlarged blood-vessels, and then waited until the parts had completely cicatrized before a second application was made. The time required for treatment by this method may be urged as an objection; but with the conscientious surgeon such an objection, when he comes to calculate the advantages of this mode of treatment, will have but little weight; and he will perhaps be quite agreeably surprised, as we were, on seeing the very small cicatrix left after the use of the caustic; and this, in cases in which the affection is seated in the face, is a matter of no small importance.

In another instance, a large aneurismal tumor, extending from the ear to the angle of the inferior maxillary bone, was much reduced in size by means of pressure with a piece of wood, carved to adapt itself over the surface, to which it was bound. Thus was a hazardous and painful operation avoided; and, in addition to the important blood-vessels involved, the individual was subject to an erysipelatous affection of the head, which interposed new obstacles to an operation.

Inflammatory Affections.—These never assume that violent and acute form on this Island that they are found to do on the continent, or in colder countries. Such as do occur, present themselves during the months of winter and spring, and are very easily controlled by depletion and the usual antiphlogistic remedies. Those cases only which are complicated with some previous disease, prove serious; but when there is but a single organ involved, the disease will yield much more readily in a native than in similar cases among the ships of the squadron.

Chronic gastritis and *enteritis* also occur, particularly during the summer and autumn. The latter, which is generally insidious in its approach, will be found very difficult of treatment among the natives, who, accustomed to the use of acrid and irritating vegetables, will rarely give that attention to diet which such cases require.

Dysentery.—In the midsummer and autumn, severe cases of acute inflammation of the mucous membrane, constituting violent forms of dysentery, prevail to some extent, but they do not now assume that violent degree that they formerly did. There is in these cases much tormina and tenesmus, with copious mucous and bloody evacuations. The accession of these cases was invariably without any premonitory symptoms; and, unless arrested by local blood-letting with leeches, they rapidly advanced to a fatal termination, the tongue being covered with a thick brown fur, and the breath being offensive. But the yellow, jaundiced appearance and highly malignant character, which this disease assumes on the coast of Africa and in the Indies, are never to be met with among the Mahonese, while those patients brought from Algiers to the military hospital at this place, presented these malignant symptoms.

Diseases of the Eye.—These in Minorca, with the exception of cataract, are found to have no higher ratio than obtains in other countries to the north, but the disease of *cataract* we met with in all ages and in all classes, to an extent far beyond anything that our experience has showed us elsewhere. *Ophthalmias* are not so severe in the accession, nor are they so violent in degree on shore, as those cases which occurred among the more robust sailors afloat. That they yielded, however, less readily to treatment, and were more serious in their consequences, we had but too many cases to prove.

Cataract.—This affection received much of our attention, having directed our care to its surgical removal; and as such operations were previously unknown here, the reports of the first cases rapidly spread, and brought many to us from all sections of the Island. Twenty-seven cases came under our observation, of which thirteen were in individuals under twenty-one years of age, one of which was congenital. The operation of extraction was performed upon seven patients; and of these, three had their sight restored, in two the vision was improved, and in the remaining two no benefit was experienced. In one of these last, an aged woman, after the removal of the lens, the incision in the cornea could not be made to unite, notwithstanding the most careful attentions and the employment of every means in our power; and ten weeks after the operation, the vitreous humors were discharged, and the eye collapsed without pain or inflammation,—a result which was, doubtless, owing to the bad habit of our patient, and the humidity of the apartments in which she was confined. The operation of couching was done three times; but in each case the lens or its capsule partially returned, and obstructed the axis of vision.

One of these patients, a beggar, after having the lens depressed in both eyes, was so much rejoiced at the restoration of his sight, by an operation attended with so little pain, that no sooner had we left his house, than he arose from his bed, went singing to a neighboring wine cellar, and congratulated himself upon his good fortune, by getting thoroughly intoxicated. The operation proved of course unsuccessful, and in consequence of his improper conduct, it was not repeated ; and, indeed, he was no ways anxious for a second operation, inasmuch as he argued that so long as he was blind, he would be certain of alms, but that with his sight restored he would be obliged to labor, and even after hard work, he would be destitute. The first case in which we extracted the lens, the individual, though aged, was in robust health. He had been deprived of vision for fifteen years; and, in this instance, the operation was followed by complete success. In another case, a priest was again enabled to discharge the duties of his holy office ; and he offered up in our behalf the most fervent prayers that we would join his faith and die a Christian, instead of a heretic, which would be sure to be followed by eternal punishment.

The case of congenital cataract was in a youth of seventeen, and the operation of keratonyxis was performed, passing a couching needle through the cornea, on its superior and outer aspect.   Upon introducing the needle through the capsule, the aqueous humor was immediately made turbid with the contents of a milky cataract ; and after the lapse of a few days, we had the satisfaction of finding that the capsule was entirely transparent, and that the entire pupil was free from every vestige of opaque matter. The delight of this boy, at seeing for the first time the light of the heavens, exceeds description, it being expressed in the most extravagant and boisterous mirth. In puncturing the capsule of the other eye, we used the needle recommended by Mr. Jacobs of Dublin ; but we found so much difficulty in passing it through the cornea, that notwithstanding the many advantages it possesses over all others, when once introduced into the chambers of the eye, we feel but little desire to use it again. The capsule of the eye last operated upon was slightly opaque on its lower surface, but still a large portion was in a proper condition for the transmission of light to the retina. The sensibility of the optic nerve was found to be much less than in its normal state, probably induced by its long inactivity. He was enabled to gaze at the sun without pain; but, as not unfrequently happens in similar cases, he was never able to fix the eye. Stars to him were invisible, yet he would watch the moon night after night with unceasing delight.

One of the first persons brought before him after the removal of the bandages, was the late lamented and gallant Commodore Hull ; and he was unable to find words to express his astonishment at seeing the

lustre of the sword, epaulettes, and the military trimmings of the naval
uniform.   The wild and involuntary rolling of his eyes would only
permit him to get a glance at the glittering gold, and he depended most
upon his cultivated sense of touch, to get fully acquainted with these
objects of his admiration.   This case, which promised so favorably,
proved ultimately of less benefit than we had anticipated ; the patient
was never able to gain any control over the motion of the eye-balls ;
they continued to roll in wild irregular movements ; and the stimulus
of the light, instead of diminishing, increased this involuntary muscular
action.

Various means were resorted to with a view to prevent these motions.
Among others, the eyes were covered with a soft leathern belt, with a
small hole directly over the axis of vision, but without any beneficial
result.   The operation was, however, so far of service to him, that he
was enabled to go about without a guide, and to perform such labors
in the fields, as would enable him to earn his bread.   On one occasion
we saw him engaged in gathering stones from a field ; he would
accurately get the direction and distance of the stone in the wild
movements of the eye ; then closing them, he would walk directly
toward it, seldom failing in placing his foot upon the object of his
search ; and in this way only was he able to perform any labor.

The frequency of cataract we could attribute only to the intense glare
of the sun, and the universal practice of white-washing.   All houses
and walls are covered with lime, and this is regularly renewed every
Saturday in the streets and front walls ; and we may here add, that
notwithstanding the poverty of the Mahonese, nowhere have we ever
met with so much cleanliness as among these people.   The dwellings
of those who often suffer from the want of food, are always in the most
perfect order, and this cardinal virtue covers many of the iniquities of
these people.

Ulcers.—From what has already been said, it may be anticipated that,
in a community so much oppressed, where the vital powers are so much
enfeebled, ulcerations are very common ; but a mere statement to that
effect would by no means convey to the reader the universal tendency
which exists to ulceration, upon the receipt of the slightest injury, and
the great difficulty that the surgeon will encounter in their treatment.
It must be acknowledged, however, that in many instances this obstinacy
and disposition to spread, are produced by the means resorted to for
their cure ; and we have often witnessed the use of the most irritating
and injurious applications.   This tendency to ulceration cannot be
attributed alone to the general impaired health of the subject ; for the
muriate of soda, which either exists at all times in the atmosphere, or
has already been deposited on the clothing or dressings, which come in
contact with the abraded surface, no doubt contributes its full share.
Injuries in the young and robust are quite as certain to terminate in
ulcers, which often extend with great rapidity, as in the aged and infirm ;
but in the treatment of the latter class of patients they will be found
the most tractable, as such persons will be more willing to submit to
perfect rest.   Indeed, without rest, they will invariably heal but slowly,
and when the ulceration is situated in the lower extremities, it will be
found almost impossible to heal them, unless the patient submits to the
horizontal posture.   With rest, however, and dressings carefully adapted
to the condition of the case, especially when aided by the internal use

of the mineral acids, the most protracted and aggravated cases were cured. The application of all ointments was uniformly of little service, and was consequently ultimately discarded; but by confining the applications to lotions, such as the solution of sulphas zinci, nitras argenti, and other astringents of this class, many cases which had resisted treatment for a long period, rapidly recovered.

A frequent consequence of these ulcerations in the lower extremities was varicose enlargement; and the operation for their obliteration, so frequently done with success in the United States, we were here unable to perform, in consequence of the inability of these people to support operations, and the great danger of phlebitis, of which we had some sad experience. We were consequently compelled to adopt a resolution in no case to resort to the knife, when there was any possibility of relief for the patient, or chances of prolonging life without it. It was only in the Mahonese that we found the patients obnoxious to these accidents after operations; for there were numerous instances in the squadron of individuals, who had been two and three years on the station, in whom recoveries from injuries and from operations took place, with the same immunity from unfavorable results, that prevails in the higher latitudes on the Continent of Europe or in North America.

We think that it has thus been clearly demonstrated that the evils, moral and physical, under which the Minorcans labor, have their origin in the endemic agency of a bad government. It is true that there are other causes in operation, as, for instance, humidity. The houses are built of a soft limestone, with very thick walls, the floors consisting always of stone and tile; and these walls and floors even in mid-summer, in consequence of their coolness, are ever covered with the moisture of the dew-point. Thus are the inmates constantly exposed to a humid atmosphere, regarded by many as a prolific source of disease,—a condition which prevails in their dwellings throughout all seasons. To this influence we were disposed to attribute, in some degree, the unsuccessful termination of several of our most important operations, particularly those upon the eye. This cause, however, is entirely subordinate to the endemic agents of a governmental origin already brought under notice; and that it has no agency in producing the increased ratio of disease, compared with the era of Cleghorn, is obvious from the fact that humidity prevailed to an equal degree, when the Island was in possession of England. Besides, when we consider that there has been no appreciable change of climatic laws, we are warranted in ascribing the chief agency in the production of the present moral and physical evils of the Minorcans to endemic causes having their origin in the administration of the public affairs of the Island.

It is thus seen that in the investigation of endemic influences, we are not to consider the agency of physical causes alone; for, equally potent with these are the social, moral, political, and intellectual conditions of a people.*

---

* As these pages are passing through the press, we discover, from the following paragraph in the National Intelligencer, that the condition of the unfortunate Mahonese has not yet been meliorated :

"HORRIBLE DESTITUTION.—We find the following from Mahon (Balearic Islands), April 21, 1843, in the *Gazette des Tribuneaux :*

' This morning our port presented a sad and strange spectacle. All the poor of

II.—MEDICAL FACULTY OF MINORCA.

The Faculty at the Balearic Islands are under the direction of the Royal Medical Junto at Madrid, without whose license no one is permitted to practise medicine or surgery within the dominions of Her Catholic Majesty; and all persons violating this law are subject to a heavy penalty which may be imposed by any of the courts. This statute, intended for the promotion of medical science, is in reality, the great obstacle in the path of the advancement of the character of the profession in Spain; for the license can always be purchased in the present crippled state of the public treasury, and the course of professional education and examinations, necessary elsewhere, is not required to procure this royal permission. The medical sub-delegate for Mahon is Dr. F. Hernandez, a gentleman of liberal education and handsome professional acquirements; and there are several other medical men here, at the head of whom stands Dr. Sancho, whose abilities and gentlemanly deportment would secure to them a high rank, wherever such qualities are appreciated; but amid the ignorance and prejudices of Mahon, their light is under a bushel. These men are eclipsed in their professional celebrity by a host of uneducated and illiterate *Medicos*, who by means of bribes have obtained the royal licence; and, dealing in the nostrums and adopting the popular prejudices of the superstitious natives, they not only monopolize the practice, but what little money is paid for medical advice, is sure to fall into their hands. At the head of these is a man of much natural tact and cleverness, and who has not only placed himself at the head of the practitioners, but has also made himself one of the leading citizens of the Island. In early life he followed the avocation of a barber, which probably initiated him into the gossip and tattle which, even in more refined and fashionable cities, form so necessary a qualification for the success of the physician. To this, he unites great moral courage; he boldly plunges into every operation, and usually succeeds in making it redound to his credit, however fatal it may have been to his patient. It is scarcely necessary to add, that this is the individual who boldly plunged the knife into the popliteal aneurism of Mr. V., before mentioned, which occasioned his premature death. The British consul exhibited to me a urinary calculus, which this surgeon had extracted, a short time before

---

the town (and they form nearly a third of the entire population), were assembled at break of day. The greater number blocked up the quay of customs, while others were swimming in the basin of the port, or were moving about in boats, of which they had taken forcible possession. Towards eight o'clock, the United States squadron, which had been here for a fortnight, and particularly two transports belonging to it, threw into the sea an immense quantity of old biscuit. The poor, who were swimming and in boats, picked them up, and some of them, so great was their hunger, ate them at the time, although saturated with sea water.

'Soon afterward the commandant of the fort came up with a considerable force and compelled the poor to retire to the interior of the town, which they did, uttering imprecations against the director of the customs. The cause of this scene was as follows: The American squadron having to renew its provision of biscuit, the commandant proposed to offer it to the municipality as a gift to the indigent. The offer was accepted; and the director of the customs was applied to for permission to land the stale biscuit free of duty. This was refused, and the commandant of the squadron, wishing to clear out his biscuit this morning, threw it into the sea, as has been stated. It was truly painful to see persons of all ages, and of both sexes, struggling in the water to catch a mouldy biscuit, and eating it at once.' "

our arrival; but unfortunately the patient, a shoemaker, had been taken from his work-bench, without any preparatory treatment, to the operating table, from which he was carried a lifeless corpse; and the stone was not removed until after his death. This individual monopolizes the most lucrative practice of the city; and with an ostentatious display of his property, throws into the background all his professional opponents. There are but few horses at Mahon, and to be able to keep one is the most conclusive evidence of being a *cavallerio*. This man accordingly makes his daily rounds to his patients, mounted. As Dean Swift says—

> It is indeed, a very sorry hack,
> But that's of course,
> For what's expected from a horse,
> With an apothecary on his back.

Carrying heavy holsters and pistols, with a golden band around his cap, this disciple of Æsculapius looks but little like an humble practitioner of the healing art.

In consequence of our introduction to surgical practice in the case of aneurism before mentioned, we were asked to do several operations, which gave us a reputation that would not have followed elsewhere. Cases flowed in upon us with great rapidity, from all directions, and in this way most of the remarkable cases came under our observation. Thus we learned much of the state of the profession, from the treatment pursued in those cases; and among these processes of cure, charms, amulets, and the superstitious influence of the Church, had a large share. The priest sells amulets to ward off and cure the tertian fevers; keeping a cross, they say, made from the fig-tree, over the heart, will have the same effect; and eating salt, while looking at the new moon, will also prevent fevers. We will not deny, however, in view of the influence of mind upon the physical frame, that the recurrence of a tertian, kept up perhaps by habit, may thus be sometimes prevented; but if these practices are not regarded by the reader as absurd in the highest degree, the two following examples will certainly rank as such.

We were called in consultation in the case of the wife of the Dutch consul,—a most estimable lady, with an interesting family,—who, at the time of our seeing her, was almost in *articulo mortis* from intussusception. In this condition, a sheep was brought into her chamber, slaughtered at the side of her bed, the omentum taken warm and reeking from it, and placed upon her abdomen,—a remedy that the native physicians assured the family would give immediate relief. On another occasion we were called to see the child of M. Orfila, a connexion of the distinguished President of the Medical Faculty of Paris, who is a native of Mahon. We found the little patient in the last stage of hydrocephalus; the pupils were dilated, and sensibility almost destroyed. On the crown of the head, a pigeon had been tied, the poor bird having been cut open and applied warm with the feathers on, the blood at the same time streaming down the little patient's face, imparting the most forbidding aspect, as it lay upon its mother's arms. The doctor, during the same time, was lecturing, in a pompous and boisterous manner, upon the virtues of a warm dove—the emblem of

3

innocence—applied to the head of an innocent babe, to draw out all the bad humors which may have collected there.

The medicines in universal repute for almost every disease which "flesh is heir to," are Morrison's pills and the purgative mixture of Le Roy. The former is for sale at every shop in the country, accompanied with a pamphlet in the Spanish language, printed in London, setting forth, in glowing colors, the incredible virtues of this panacea; all of which is readily believed by the ignorant, who swallow these pills without limit. Many instances of their injurious, nay fatal consequences, came under our observation. Among these was the case of a paymaster in the Spanish army, who, after six years of active service in the field, during the civil war, reached Mahon, worn down and exhausted by the incessant labors and exposures of the camp. Immediately after his arrival, he was placed on the use of Morrison's pills, taking large doses of them daily. The excessive purging increased the prostration under which he had previously labored, and mortification took place in one foot, which, after great sufferings, came off at the ankle. In another case, of an old friar who had suffered for years from asthma, these pills were directed in immense quantities, which were increased as he grew worse. At length, unable to take the pills, they were dissolved and administered in solution; and we were informed by M. Sintès, a most respectable druggist, that within six days he had taken more than five hundred pills,—a cause quite sufficient to put a period to his existence. Whatever good these pills may have accomplished in England, the evil that they have occasioned in this little Island will more than counterbalance; and it is much to be regretted, that such remedies are sent abroad, with all the emblazonry of noble patronage at home, only to deal misery and death among the unfortunate and too credulous, who suppose that, because they come from Britain, where the medical profession are known to possess so much ability, they must necessarily be useful for all the diseases for which they are recommended. Upon the mercenary authors of this wholesale murder rests a fearful and a dreadful responsibility, and although they may escape human laws, yet a retributive justice awaits them hereafter.

Our practice being in every case gratuitous, it soon became extensive; and we rejoiced to have it in our power to assist, by medical advice, the large number who were suffering from the want of it. But when fully engaged in the midst of our career, we were officially notified by most formidable bulletins from the medical sub-delegate, that, in consequence of our not having a licence from the Government at Madrid, we must for the future desist in our practice. At the same time, we were informed by him, that it was, on his part, only a matter of form, which he was compelled to adopt in virtue of his office, and that we might continue to render our services as heretofore. He assured us that there would be no further proceedings in the case; and accordingly, we continued to prescribe and operate whenever necessary; and in every operation of importance, a majority of the faculty, with the medical students of the town, were always present. In a short time, however, we were duly ordered to appear before the chief-justice of the Island, and answer to a long series of charges for operating and rendering medical advice, in the various cases duly mentioned, after having been notified by the proper officer to desist.

Trial by jury is here unknown, but fortunately the judge, before whom the case was brought, was our friend in return for some small service rendered to a member of his family. These proceedings at court were conducted with an ingenuity which would have been creditable to a Philadelphia lawyer, or some of the gentlemen of the long robe at Westminster Hall. We will, therefore, mention one or two of the most important points. The first case mentioned in the indictment was for having extracted a cataract from the eye of Mr. Escudera, in the presence of some ten or twelve of the citizens of Mahon; and although all these gentlemen were present, yet the fact of the operation was not proved to the satisfaction of the court. One did not look on while operating, another did not see the lens extracted, a third did not know the day of the month on which it was done, and a fourth stated that it was in the afternoon and not in the morning, as set forth in the indictment; all of which was deemed sufficient to acquit us of the charge. During the investigation, the judge received several abusive and threatening anonymous letters, the authorship of which was attributed to one of the native physicians, who, upon being charged with it, plead "not guilty." The writing was disguised, but, unluckily for the author, the very fact that he did not find an education necessary to the art of physic, served for his conviction; for, as the letter contained many errors of orthography, the judge directed him to write a copy of the letter as it was dictated to him in court; and, when compared with the anonymous letter, unfortunately for him, every error was found to correspond precisely, notwithstanding the handwriting was entirely different.

The decision of the court was in our favor, and the cost, amounting to forty dollars, was ordered to be paid by the Medical Association of the place; but this event was followed by an open declaration of war on the part of the united faculty, who drove us from the field by the following formidable document, through the hands of O. Rich, Esq., U. S. Consul, and Commodore Isaac Hull :—

" Subdelegation of the Medical Junto at Mahon.

"SIR,—It has been repeatedly complained of to the Medical Subdelegate of Mahon, that you gave and still give advice, and practice as a Physician and Surgeon among the citizens of Her Catholic Majesty's dominions, without the Royal licence. You are, therefore, hereby notified, positively and peremptorily, to discontinue all such practices for the future; and you are not permitted to perform the functions of a Physician or Surgeon to any other individuals than the Anglo-American citizens of your own country.

"I kiss your hand.

"F. HERNANDEZ, *Medical Subdelegate.*

"J. M. FOLTZ, *Surgeon U. S. Navy.*

After the reception of this missile, we declined giving our advice to such as applied for it; but a few days after, a child was brought to us from Barcelona, in Spain, with club feet, which was of a proper age and in an excellent condition for an operation. At the same time, a lieutenant of the Spanish army applied for aid, with a permission from the governor for us to prescribe in his case, which we offered cheerfully to do, on condition that permission would be also given to operate on the child; but this his excellency refused to grant. Still desirous to relieve the child, which had undergone the dangers of a voyage at sea for the purpose of having this operation done, we proposed to operate on board one of the ships of war in the harbor; but the father, a British subject and a man of some property, prudently declined, as he was convinced, should we operate after the positive refusal of the governor, that the opportunity would be gladly seized upon to impose on him a heavy fine. The child was, therefore, taken to Marseilles, at the hazard of another voyage at sea, to have an operation done, which could have been performed here in two or three minutes.

We have been particular in detailing these cases, as they will not only give a correct idea of the condition of the medical profession in Spain, but will also apprise the reader of the oppression of the government. The only hospital or charitable institution at Mahon is an hospital for foundlings, which is liberally endowed, having at this time about one hundred names upon its register entitled to its charities, among whom are twenty-seven children. Every child deposited here can ever after claim the shelter of the institution; and, although usually placed out to masters as soon as they reach a proper age, yet they ever look to this establishment as their home in after life. There is throughout the Island no dispensary for the distribution of medicines to the poor; and, so far as we could judge, there is but little charity to them from the medical men. They are, indeed, compelled by their own wants to ask some remuneration for their services, insisting usually upon some fee, and being willing to take the most trifling amount rather than to go away empty-handed. As we were ordered, shortly after these doctors' quarrels, for service afloat, the little ill-will occasioned for the moment was soon " in the deep bosom of the ocean buried." We shall, indeed, ever rejoice to hear of their individual and united prosperity, for there are among them many of whom we shall ever have the most agreeable and pleasing recollections, and we shall pray that the causes which have occasioned their present humble position may speedily be removed.

III.—FRENCH MILITARY HOSPITAL ON THE ISLE DE LOS REYOS.

Near the centre of the harbor of Mahon is the Isle de los Reyos,— a small island on which a large naval hospital was erected, in 1796, by Sir William Burnett, the present distinguished physician in chief of the British navy. This harbor, at that time, when the supremacy of the seas was contested with England by the combined navies of France and Spain, was the great naval depot of Great Britain in this sea; and it was from this port that Toulon was kept in blockade under Lords Nelson and Collingwood. Fort St. Philip, at the entrance of the port, was then one of the most formidable fortifications in the world, which, however, was blown up and destroyed before the Island was surrendered. The hospital erected for the use of the British fleet is still in a good state of preservation, consisting of two parallel ranges of wards, which would comfortably accommodate six hundred patients. These two wings are connected at either end by ranges of buildings, intended for the officers of the establishment, with the necessary offices of such an institution; and throughout, the buildings are well adapted for the purposes for which they were intended. During the summer of 1835, the cholera made its appearance in our squadron, and a portion of the building was appropriated for the use of the sick; but since then they have not been occupied.

The protracted wars in Algeria, where that indomitable chief, Abd-el-kader, has year after year subverted all the grand projects of the army of France, had filled the hospitals at Algiers to overflowing; and the French government applied for the use of the hospital at Mahon, for such of the sick as were able to be transported to this island,—an application which was promptly granted.

We visited Algiers in the summer of 1839, the first year of the war against the Bedouin chief, at which time the total number of troops in the colony was forty-five thousand. Since then, the number of troops has at various times exceeded seventy thousand, and disastrous as these campaigns have been, the number destroyed by their formidable enemies is but a fraction of those who fell victims to the climate. As nearly as we could ascertain from credible sources of information, there has been an average of three thousand deaths among the troops from dysentery and fever every summer, since the commencement of the war. When it is remembered that these troops all leave France in perfect health, and that they remain but a short time in Africa, it will be seen that this army has suffered dreadfully. Dysentery and fevers annually sweep their ranks, and not only are the hospitals crowded to overflowing with the sick and dying, but even the highways are strewed with them; and such are yearly their privations and sufferings, that none but a nation with the highest enthusiasm for military glory and renown, could endure them. The total number sick in the hospital at Algiers at the period of our visit, was near three thousand. These were accommodated in three hospitals; one was within the town, containing about five hundred, the other two were without the walls of the city, being large, spacious, and well supplied with every necessary. One stands on the east, the other on the west side of the town, constituting series of extensive stone buildings, one story high, erected for the cavalry of the Dey; but they have been converted into military hospitals, for which, in this warm climate, they are peculiarly adapted.

In the winter of 1839 and '40, a commission, consisting of a physician, a surgeon, and an officer of engineers, arrived at Mahon, and placed the hospital and apartments at the quarantine in a condition to receive the sick. The buildings throughout were placed in perfect order, and between four and five hundred beds were arranged for the reception of such invalids as could endure the fatigues of transportation from Algiers, a distance of two hundred and fifty miles; and early in the summer, every bed was occupied. As soon as sufficiently recovered, they were sent on to Toulon, and their places filled by weekly arrivals from the seat of war. Nine-tenths of these patients suffered from dysentery and enteritis, and very many died on their passage or immediately after their arrival. Such was the desire of all once more to see "*la belle France,*" that many, in their dying moments, piteously implored to be sent on board the steamers, which were especially arranged for their comfort, convinced that only to leave the shores of Africa would ensure their recovery; and we were informed by the medical officers, that recoveries did in very many cases take place, which had been hopeless, and in which all attempts at a cure by any other means would have been unavailing. Such were the operations of hope, and of the love of home.

3*

upon the minds of these enthusiastic and gallant soldiers; and there can exist no doubt but that the establishment of this hospital was the means of saving many a valuable life.

The medical part of the hospital was under the charge of M. Hutin, and the surgical under that of M. Jourdan, both gentlemen of the highest professional attainments; and these principals were assisted by a corps of about thirty assistants, than whom no men could have been more devoted to their duties; and it is with much pleasure that we are able to record our testimony in favor of the humanity and kindness with which the sufferings and wants of these soldiers of France were administered to by their medical attendants. As further proof of the military character and honor of this chivalrous nation, we will mention that every medical officer, in addition to his oath of office, makes a solemn and public pledge of his honor, that in every case in which aid is required, he will render it with kindness and humanity; and faithfully did those at the military hospital at Mahon redeem their pledge.

We regret our inability to give the correct number of admissions, discharges, and deaths. The first and last were, however, very great, the mortality being evidently due to the malignancy of the diseases acquired in one of the most insalubrious parts of the globe, in which the most efficient medical treatment would be of little avail.

In the treatment, the influence of Broussais' school was very manifest; leeches and enemata, with mucilaginous and demulcent drinks, formed the basis of all remediate measures; and this treatment in recent cases, or in a less aggravated form of disease than was here presented, would doubtless have been very efficient. Having ourselves encountered this form of malignant febrile disease in its very hot-bed, at Batavia, in the East Indies, where the progress was so rapid that it often proved fatal within forty-eight and seventy-two hours from the time of the accession, we found that the only safety for the patient consisted in an energetic and vigorous treatment; and this disease of Africa presented many of the peculiar symptoms which were met with in the disease as presented in India, particularly in the derangement of the functions of the skin and liver, in which the prompt but judicious use of the lancet and mercury were loudly demanded. For the successful treatment of this disease in the East, we were indebted to the invaluable work of Dr. James Johnson on tropical climates; and much esteemed as that excellent work is in Europe and the United States, it is to the practitioner in intertropical climates only that its great merits can be known. From what we witnessed in the hospitals of Algiers, as well as that at Mahon, we were convinced of a similarity as regards the etiology, and we would have consequently rejoiced to have seen the same energetic treatment which we had found so effectual elsewhere pursued in these cases. In the violent diseases of warm countries, where the system is exposed to malaria and miasm, their progress is always rapid; and even in those milder cases, where the patient himself suffers but little, he usually survives a mere wreck, with premature old age and debility; all of which might have been prevented by a bold and active treatment in the early stages of the disease.

Various proceedings on the part of the French excited the suspicions of the Spanish government, and it did not escape the observation of that vigilant officer, Colonel Fitzgerald, her Britannic majesty's consul at Mahon, that France was looking toward an occupation of this group of islands, as her first step upon the explosion of the Eastern question, which at that time engaged the attention of all Europe. Careful surveys were made of the harbor, and the elevation and distance of the surrounding hills were accurately made by the French engineers; but, notwithstanding the care evidently taken not to excite observation, these measures were speedily followed by an order from Madrid, for the French to evacuate the hospital on La isle de los Reyos. This was effected in the spring of 1841; and it subsequently appeared, from the declaration of M. Jaubert, in the French Chambers, who held a situation in the ministry under the Thiers administration, that the cabinet had actually determined to occupy the Balearic Islands, as her first movement in the war. To this England would, doubtless, have interposed her protest,—a measure which would have been hailed with delight by the oppressed and helpless inhabitants of this valuable Island, with whom a change of government,—the only panacea for their evils, political and social, moral and physical,—forms the subject of their daily prayers.

IV.—STATISTICS OF THE UNITED STATES' NAVAL HOSPITAL AT MAHON.

At the period of entering upon the duties of hospital surgeon to the Mediterranean squadron, the force consisted of one hundred and sixty guns, with eighteen hundred men, under the command of Commodore Isaac Hull, with the Ohio (eighty guns) flag-ship. Subsequently a forty-four gun frigate joined the force, which increased the number of men to twenty-two hundred. The crowded state of ships of war, at all times, renders the situation of the sick on board extremely uncomfortable; and when the number of invalids is great, they materially interfere with the duties of the ship. At the same time that they impair her efficiency, the wet decks and exposure to atmospheric vicissitudes, materially retard their recovery. An hospital was therefore established at this port,—the depot for the squadron,—for the treatment of such cases of disease and accidents (to which sailors are peculiarly subject), as cannot receive the necessary comforts and attendance on board ship.

The building appropriated for the purpose was a large dwelling, situated on the borders of the town, and sufficiently extensive comfortably to accommodate about forty patients; but we have had more than sixty within its walls at the same time, embracing, however, many cases which could be crowded together without inconvenience to one another. Three weeks before our arrival, twenty-two invalids from the hospital, including one officer, sailed for the United States. Of these, seven had affections of the chest, five chronic enteritis, two stricture, two epilepsy, three rheumatism, one syphilitic iritis, and two were superannuated. Two died on the passage home. On the 17th of August, nine patients entered the hospital, who had just been admitted to pratique after twenty days' quarantine. They had last been upon the coast of Syria and Egypt, where at this season, the plague is always found; but which has never made its appearance on board our ships of war, notwithstanding they cruise in the Levant annually. Five of these cases had affections of the alimentary canal, one had a fracture, one phthisis, one syphilis, and one rheumatism. The case of phthisis was a native of New Grenada, having apparently been a long time in bad health, and having suffered, when young, from the epidemic fevers of the Magdalena river.   When admitted he was much emaciated; he had copious expectoration of pus, hectic, and night sweats.   Our treatment could only be palliative, and in the third week of his admission, he éxpired.   Upon a post-mortem examination, tubercles were not only found in the lungs, but also in the meninges of the brain.

September 6th.   Fourteen were admitted after having passed the summer cruising in the Archipelago.   Nine of these cases were chronic diarrhœa, the consequence of dysentery, which had prevailed to some extent, but in a mild form, during the season.   Two had ulcers, one secondary syphilis, one epilepsy, and one coxalgia.   These cases presented nothing remarkable in their character, nor were they more difficult in treatment than such cases usually are in seamen; for they, be it understood, rejoice in availing themselves of every opportunity to "weather the doctor," and resort to every expedient to procure liquor and indulge in the worst of dissipation, notwithstanding it is always at the expense of much suffering and not unfrequently even at the risk of life.   As the poor sailor has but little to live for, often an outcast from friends and home, a wanderer upon the wide world, he is best satisfied, when disease and death approach, if his suffering can be abbreviated. We have ourselves witnessed many cases, considered incurable by the patient himself, in which, with the recklessness peculiar to a seaman, he has indulged in dissipation with a view of accelerating death; and from this indulgence he can be protected only by the unceasing vigilance of the officers.

A majority of the admissions were from diseases of the intestinal canal, which naval practitioners find among the most frequent, as well as among the most unmanageable of the diseases of seamen; and this tendency to gastric disease, especially in hot climates, is doubtless produced by the indigestible diet to which they are confined at sea.   This follows from the fact, that the salt provisions are frequently kept years before they are served out, which, with the beans, ships' duff, and large quantity of spirits formerly issued, produce those severe forms of gastric affections, as well as dyspepsia, to which sailors are peculiarly subject.   In the last named disease, the most judicious and careful treatment will be of little avail, so long as the patient is confined on board ship; but if a change to a residence on shore is made, with a mild farinaceous diet, more will be effected in a few weeks, than any treatment on board.   When ulceration had taken place in the mucous membrane, which will be found to be the case in a majority of instances, the mineral astringents are found most effectual; and at the head of these remedies stands, agreeably to our experience, the acetate of lead, in doses of from one to two grains, twice a day, in combination with one-eighth of a grain of opium.   This we have repeatedly known to cure the most inveterate cases supervening upon the severe forms of the dysentery of the tropics.   The sulphate of copper, in doses of one-sixteenth to one-eighth of a grain, combined with opium or lactucarium, we have also used with benefit; but a careful attention to diet will be found the most important matter in such cases, to which, the use of enemata of cold water or a simple infusion of sem. lini will be useful adjuvants.   No article of the materia medica, have we seen do as much good, in those chronic affections of the intestines, as the acetate of lead properly administered. Care should be taken that the preparation contain no carbonate of lead, from which alone unpleasant consequences are to be apprehended.

Case of Hemiplegia.—One of the most important cases under treatment at this time, was that of assistant-surgeon Van Wyck, who was affected with hemiplegia. As we had but a short time previously met with several of the cases of Mr. Turnbull, in London, in which the use of the strychnine was attended with benefit, we eagerly embraced this opportunity of prescribing this article; and from the youth and general good health of the patient, we entered upon the treatment, sanguine of success. The patient was twenty-one years of age, and had just entered the navy after a collegiate course, in which he had carried away the highest honors; and from his devotion to his profession, he promised much future usefulness. Within twenty-four hours of sailing from New York, he was seized with paralysis of the left side, which also deprived him of the powers of articulation. Three months elapsed from the time of being paralyzed, until he came under our care. From the time of the attack he had been subject to violent epileptic convulsions, which returned periodically, at intervals of about a fortnight. For this he had been copiously bled, which for the future was avoided as much as possible; and it was found that arresting the circulation in the extremities by means of a tourniquet, would seldom fail to put a stop to the convulsions, which is a method of treatment that we have practised with much success in the epilepsy of seamen,—a class of men who are very obnoxious to this disease. We have recently seen it mentioned in the European journals, that pressure upon the carotids will seldom fail to arrest epileptic convulsions; and from the benefit which we have so frequently witnessed, from pressure upon the arteries of the extremities, we could confidently anticipate the best results from interrupting the circulation in the carotids, in those cases in which there is so great a determination to the brain, as frequently to cause the production of lesions and effusions. The strychnine was ordered in solution, commencing with one-sixteenth of a grain, *ter in die,* and the paralyzed side was bathed once a day with a solution of nux vomica. The dose was gradually increased until one-third of a grain was taken, when spasms and involuntary muscular contractions took place in the paralyzed limbs. This manifestation of the influence of the medicine was hailed as a favorable symptom, and its use was now diligently persevered in, with the effect of increasing the spasmodic action to a great extent; but no additional voluntary motion was acquired. At the termination of eight weeks' use of the strychnine, as the convulsions became very violent, and the symptoms presented indications that the system was suffering from the medicine, its use was discontinued; and hereupon, these unpleasant symptoms gradually disappeared. At intervals, for several months, the strychnine was ordered in various forms, and in smaller quantities, but without any favorable result. A seton in the nape of the neck was of service; and after restoring his general health, he ultimately embarked for the United States in charge of his relatives, who encountered all the difficulties of a voyage to the Mediterranean, to restore him again to the family circle. In this case, as well as in the numerous instances in which the strychnine was administered among the natives, the favorable consequences did not follow which were met with in the hands of Mr. Turnbull.

Upon the termination of the quarter ending the 30th of September, twenty-two patients were under treatment in the hospital, including three officers. Of these, five had affections of the chest, nine of the intestinal canal, two syphilis, one fracture, one epilepsy, two rheumatism, one coxalgia, and one ulcer. One patient had died during the quarter from tubercular phthisis.

For the quarter ending the 31st of December, 1839, sixty-two had been admitted. Of these, thirty-one were cases of itch, in boys, who were immediately transferred to the hospital, to guard against a propagation of the disease in crowded ships. This affection is one which is very prevalent among seamen,—a liability attributable in a great degree to their diet; and, as may be anticipated, difficulties are presented in its cure, which are seldom or never encountered in private practice. Five of the cases resisted the administration of sulphur externally and internally; but the eruption speedily disappeared under the use of an ointment of the iodide of iron, with small alterative doses of the proto-iodide of mercury, prohibiting at the same time the use of stimulating animal food. There is in this disease unquestionably much less liability to its attack in those who have previously suffered from it; and in not a few, it observes the law which obtains among many of the exanthemata, of securing an immunity from a second attack in the same individual; and we have met with many cases of serious organic affections, the development of which could be distinctly traced to a severe attack of psora. Of the remaining cases, eleven were affections of the chest, of which two proved fatal within the quarter; three were fractures, one dislocation, one paralysis, one aneurism, one syphilis, and one rheumatism.

Case of Aneurism.—The case of aneurism was in the person of an aged quarter-gunner, who, from his long and useful services, had strong claims upon our careful attentions, but who proved a most ungovernable and unmanageable patient. He was fifty-five years of age, and for twelve months previous to his admission, had suffered much from violent palpitations of the heart, and recently, a tumor had made its appearance beneath the left clavicle, which pulsated strongly. In the umbilical region, there was also a very perceptible enlargement, which not only pulsated strongly when pressed upon in a line with the artery, but communicated the same throbbing sensation when elevated from the spine by lateral pressure, which, as the patient was much emaciated, could be easily effected; and it was from this abdominal tumor that he suffered most inconvenience. His only complaint was from the "*thumping amidship,*" as he expressed it. Having witnessed the most happy results from the strict enforcement of the treatment of Valsalva among the native Minorcans, we were desirous of pursuing the same course in this case; and for many days, and even weeks, when closely watched, he confined himself to his bed, taking no other food than the most mild and unirritating diet, while Withering's infusion of digitalis was administered to the fullest extent that his system would allow. Under this course he was much improved, which promised at least to prolong his life, and pass it comparatively without pain; but, in the midst of this nursing, he would at midnight leave his bed, scale the walls, and without his clothing rush to the first grogshop. Here he would drink, quarrel and fight, as long as he was able to stand; and when overcome by his exertions, he would be brought back to the hospital, to undergo another course of arrow-root and digitalis. When intoxicated, his exertions were powerful, and it was frequently necessary to resort to the use of the strait-jacket, during his *furor ;* and at these times, the action of the heart and throbbing in the aneurismal tumors were so violent, as to occasion great apprehension of an immediate rupture. In this situation, it was necessary to bleed him freely ; and such was the condition of his fluids, that the blood contained but little coloring matter, and from the scarification, after the use of cups, serum would continue to flow until arrested by a compress. This course continued for many months, until his final return to the United States. We were equally astonished at the great strength manifested by him when under the influence of liquor, and that the case did not prove fatal during some one of his excesses. After each debauch, when perhaps scarcely able to raise his head, he would say that he felt much better ; and if we would only give him a little more rum, he would be sure to get well. Had our patient joined the "tee-totallers," it would have been of more service to him than all our medicine and advice.

Very many cases are brought to the hospital occurring among the seamen when on shore, during their liberty ; and these cases are often severe injuries, received in their quarrels with one another, or with the Spaniards on shore. In the latter case, the injuries are often of a very serious character. Unacquainted with the use of the fist, the Spaniards, in these encounters, fly in every direction from before the sailor ; but, carefully storing up this defeat, and never permitting an opportunity of revenge to pass by, they clandestinely put a knife into the back of poor Jack, who is equally ignorant of their mode of fighting. Two of the cases of fracture admitted, occurred on shore, one of them being a fracture of the lower jaw, from a blow with a stone, causing much injury to the soft parts ; and it was only after some months of much suffering, during which it was found necessary to extract two of the molar teeth, that the patient recovered. Very many are brought to the hospital in an extreme state of intoxication and delirium tremens,—a disease which is encountered in naval practice, to an extent unknown in private life. Nowhere in life, can so great a change be seen in the condition of men, as in the crew of a ship of war mustered on the quarter deck to receive permission for liberty on shore, and the appearance of the same men twenty-four or forty-eight hours after. In the former case, they are all ruddy, hardy, happy chaps, in their neat sailor's dress, with ribands flying, and their pockets filled with more money than they can properly spend during their short run on shore. In this state they land for the purpose of having " a good jolly drunk." At the termination of the leave, which never exceeds forty-eight hours, they are gathered together by the officers, often without hats, jackets, or shoes ; their eyes blackened, and the few clothes on them in strips and tatters ; and it is often necessary to hoist them on board in the same way as a portion of a ship's cargo.

We rejoice to have it in our power to say, that nowhere has the temperance cause done so much good as among seamen. Every inducement is, indeed, held out by giving to the temperate a portion of each month's wages and frequent liberty. By holding out this inducement to all who will abstain from drink, and by this alone, may the whole character of the seaman be revolutionized. After the liberty of a crew of five hundred men, the surgeon will have more cases of delirium tremens under his care than would be encountered for a long period in private practice; but the disease is very easily treated among seamen, as we are always able to prevent a further indulgence, which so frequently thwarts the best directed efforts in private practice. During our experience of more than twelve years in the navy, but a single fatal case from this disease has come under our observation, and in that instance it was associated with hæmoptysis.   The remedies these cases are emetics and opium, and when there is much arterial excitement, venesection.   The first two, however, are the means upon which we chiefly rely.   The use of emetics in this disease is more loudly called for among seamen than in any other class of persons; for, no sooner do they reach the shore than they commence eating and drinking the richest food and the worst of fruits and drinks that come in their way, until their stomachs are filled to repletion.   In this condition, fluids alone can find entrance, and care is taken to renew the supplies so long as they are able to keep on their feet; and in this state of insensibility, they are brought to us for treatment.   Here, a dose of ipecacuanha will be of more importance than any other remedy; and he will disgorge a mess sufficient to be a surfeit for any man.   No sooner is he relieved from his burden, than sensibility and motion are restored; he opens his eyes in a furious, wild delirium, with the " horrors," and calls for something to drink.   In this stage, a glass of hot toddy, with twenty-five drops of tr. opii, will seldom fail to tranquillize him; and a few doses more will induce a sound sleep, from which he will awake ready for another cruize either at sea or on shore.   When this treatment does not succeed, and there is much delirium with a full pulse, venesection should be resorted to.   After this, the administration of opium and asafœtida, in large doses, will be sure to tranquillize the nervous system, and procure a profound sleep, which last is, in all cases, the best restorer of exhausted nature.

During the quarter, seventy-one were returned on board ship for duty, three died, and two were discharged the service at their own request.   Thus thirty-nine were left under treatment on the 1st of January, 1840, of whom five were officers; and these last had their quarters in private dwellings, as the hospital had been too much crowded, during the quarter, to allow them the necessary comforts.

For the first quarter of 1840, thirty-seven were admitted.   Of these, eighteen had affections of the chest, among whom were several young men, who had the most copious hæmoptysis, without having suffered from any premonitory symptoms, indicative of disease of the lungs.   In one case, a young man brought on shore as an attendant upon the sick, was seized with the most violent hæmorrhage, which assumed a periodical form, returning daily for a fortnight, followed by hectic fever and the suppuration of vomicæ, and within six weeks of the attack, the case terminated fatally.   On post-mortem examination, tubercles were revealed throughout the whole pulmonary tissue.

At this season of the year much rain falls, particularly at night, when it descends in torrents; the prevailing north-west winds are cold and disagreeable; and although the thermometer seldom falls as low as 48°, yet the cold is much more unpleasant, and we suffer more from it, than when the thermometer is at the freezing point in the United States.

The records of the squadron prove that, notwithstanding the lauded salubrity of the Mediterranean and the advantages to be derived from it by the pulmonary invalid, this island, at least, possesses none of these immunities. On the contrary, all who were predisposed to pulmonary disease, or were of a tubercular diathesis, were sure to have the latent disease developed; and the only deaths which, up to this period, had occurred at the hospital, with two exceptions, were from phthisis. Seven of the patients received were cases of rheumatism, two of fracture, two of scrofula (one of which was accompanied with an inflammation of the knee joint, which terminated in anchylosis), one of nyctalopia (which continued to resist all treatment until the patient's departure for the United States), and one of hepatitis. The remaining five were not such as to require particular notice.

Abscess of the Liver.—The case of hepatitis was the consequence of an attack of fever on the coast of Africa, which was followed by great derangement of the hepatic functions; the skin had remained dry, parched and yellow, with much gastric disturbance. With the approach of cold weather, hepatitis set in, the right hypochondriac region being much enlarged and very painful, without the ability to bear the slightest pressure. After the inflammatory stage passed by, rigors, loss of sensibility over the inflamed part, with great prostration and discoloration, indicated the occurrence of suppuration in the liver; and in this stage of the case, we contemplated making an incision into the abscess, as fluctuation could be detected by a careful examination; but we were deterred from the operation by the great prostration and unfavorable condition of the patient. The pulse was quick, tense and frequent, with coldness of the surface and of the extremities, attended with copious serous alvine evacuations. After remaining in this condition for several days, the hepatic abscess burst through the right lung during a fit of coughing, and discharged an immense quantity of bloody pus. His strength was now supported by nutritious diet and drinks, by means of which his life was prolonged until the tenth day after the bursting of the abscess. Upon examination, it was found that the entire liver had been much enlarged; the right lobe formed an immense abscess, which had suppurated by an irregular opening through the diaphragm into the lung; and the entire convex surface of the liver was firmly united to the parietes of the abdomen. Had an artificial opening been made, or had the ulceration been external, there could have been no effusion into the abdominal cavity in consequence of this adhesion; and notwithstanding the almost positive certainty of death, we regretted having not plunged a scalpel into the abscess, as that was the only possibility of saving life. In such cases, a desperate and energetic effort is the only means left for the exercise of humanity. The other viscera of the abdomen were in a comparatively healthy state, notwithstanding being almost in contact with the extensively diseased liver.

A case of *secondary syphilis*, in a petty officer, which had for more than a twelvemonth resisted every method of treatment, came under our care. The mercurial and anti-mercurial methods of treatment had each been tried, without any benefit; and in this state, with extensive ulcerations in the fauces, venereal eruptions, with a slow and gradual progression of the disease, we resolved upon the course of fumigations recommended by Mr. Abernethy. Frictions with the mercurial

4

ointment and the internal administration of the protiodide of mercury had been practised, but without any favorable results. One pound of the protochloride of hydrargyrum was washed with a diluted mixture of ammonia, and the precipitate dried; and with this he was carefully fumigated each alternate day, for twenty days. After each fumigation, the whole surface was covered with the impalpable powder of the oxide of mercury, and the same clothes were worn throughout next the skin. This course was followed by much febrile excitement, loss of sleep and appetite, with nervous tremors throughout the whole system, indicating the action of the metal, without any of the specific effects in producing salivation; and, at the same time, the ulcers in the throat, as well as the eruption, assumed a more aggravated and unhealthy aspect. The mercurial fumigations were of course discontinued, the patient confined to a warm room, and the decoction of sarsaparilla ordered. Guaiacum in large doses was afterwards administered, which, with low diet and care, after a lapse of three months, finally conquered this obstinate case.

The remaining cases did not present any remarkable feature, notwithstanding many of them were of the most serious character. In these last, our only efforts could be directed toward relieving the most urgent symptoms, and rendering the remainder of the patient's life comfortable. This duty can, in truth, always be performed with pleasure, if the subject is an old sailor, who has faithfully served his country,— one who, from the nature of his calling, is a wanderer upon the wide world, without friends or home,— and who, whatever may be his failings, is never ungrateful for services rendered when prostrated by disease.

The total number under treatment, for the last three months, was seventy-six. Of these, forty-one were returned to duty cured, and two died, leaving in the hospital, on the 31st of March, thirty-three still under treatment. Of these last, a majority were incurable cases, and were designated as such in the quarterly report to the commander of the forces.

On the 12th April, a survey was held upon the patients in the hospital, and twenty-two cases were pronounced proper subjects to be sent to the United States as invalids. They were accordingly embarked in a store-ship, on the 18th of April, under charge of the Surgeon of the Fleet, Dr. Ticknor, the present able surgeon of the naval hospital at New York, to whom on this occasion we would express our kind acknowledgments, as well as to his successor, Surgeon Thos. Williamson, whose reputation in the service is too well established to require anything to be said in this place. Of the twenty-two invalids sent home, seven had affections of the chest, three rheumatism, two stricture, one aneurism, one nyctalopia, one anchylosis of the knee-joint, one insanity, and the remainder came under the class of general impaired health and advanced age. This number included two officers. Since the 1st of the month, one had died and five were returned to duty, leaving, after the departure of the incurables, but five patients which were considered cases that would yield to the treatment and comforts of the hospital.

Nearly one year had elapsed since our arrival at Mahon; and throughout this period we had suffered much from intermittent fever, brought on, in the first instance, by exposure to an intensely hot sun, during an excursion into the interior of the Island immediately after our arrival. These paroxysms were easily checked by quinine; but, upon the slightest exposure, they were sure to return. It was, therefore, with much pleasure, that we embraced an opportunity which offered, to cruise at sea during the summer months, which were passed in the Adriatic and Archipelago.

The hospital, in the mean time, was in charge of Assistant Surgeon Sinclair; and upon our return to Mahon, on the 5th of November, from the coast of Asia Minor, it was found that there had been nine admitted during our absence. Five had been returned to duty cured, one having been operated upon for hydrocele, and one had died from phthisis, leaving, at the time of our resuming the charge of the hospital, eight patients under treatment. After the usual quarantine, we received twenty-one into the hospital, all of whom had been cruising to the East; eight of them having passed the summer on the coasts of Syria and Egypt, at that time the seat of war. Eleven of these cases were affections of the stomach and bowels, five of the chest, two were cases of fever, one of ophthalmia, and two of injuries. One of the sick who was advanced in years, and was in bad health at the time of his arrival on the station, died on the eleventh day of his admission into the hospital, of disease of the lungs.

Case of Tetanus.—One of those admitted in consequence of an injury was a carpenter's mate, who had a nail run into his foot eight weeks before coming to the hospital. Symptoms of tetanus followed the accident, for which the incision had been freely enlarged and cauterized, and the usual remedies administered with only temporary relief. His case terminated in chronic tetanus, the only instance of that disease which has ever fallen under our observation. The patient was twenty-six years of age, temperate in his habits, and at the time of the accident in good health. The only relief he had heretofore obtained was from the use of large quantities of opium, to the extent of a complete saturation of the system, but as soon as the operation of the narcotic would subside the spasms invariably returned. The treatment was commenced at the hospital, by again freely laying open the puncture in the sole of the foot, and dividing the nerves in the vicinity. The base of the wound was then covered with the nitras argenti, and suppuration encouraged by cataplasms. This operation, which was attended with much pain, was followed by a copious suppuration, which was carefully kept up; and the part, at the same time, was washed with a syringe, in the hope that it would bring away any particles of metal which might remain, causing the irritation. After several weeks, the wound healed, forming apparently a sound and healthy cicatrix, but the tetanic symptoms remained with their usual severity. Spasms occurred almost daily, inducing violent opisthotonos, the muscles of the jaw being at the same time affected. During the intermission from spasm, the patient was enabled to sit up. His general health became very good, suffering only from constipation produced by the large quantities of opium which he was in the habit of taking. From the habitual use of this narcotic, his system gradually lost the susceptibility to its influence; and hence the lactucarium and stramonium were from time to time substituted. A mercurial course was determined upon; and being profusely salivated, the spasms became much less violent, and of less frequent occurrence, but upon the subsidence of the ptyalism they again returned with their former severity. Three months after his admission into the hospital, his foot was without pain or swelling, and his general health had much improved, but there was still, at intervals of two or three days, a regular recurrence of the pain and spasms. Epispastics were applied over the spinal column, and as soon as healed were renewed, but no relief followed. Iron, bark, and quinine had also been prescribed with the same want of success. Eight months after the injury, he was returned as an invalid to the United States, and here he arrived after a long and boisterous passage, almost worn down by his protracted and intense sufferings.

Small Pox.—One of the officers, admitted this quarter, had an eruption on the face, which had suddenly made its appearance. Two days after his admission it proved to be variola, and within a few days two other cases in the hospital were developed. In consequence of this, the hospital, which is situated in the town, was immediately placed in quarantine. Health officers were ordered to guard it, and intercourse with the inmates was strictly prohibited. These cases from the hospital were sent to the quarantine buildings, at the entrance of the harbor, and placed in charge of Passed Assistant Surgeon Malcolm Smith. The number of cases within a few days increased to eleven, all from the frigate Brandywine, which had recently arrived from Lisbon. In three of these cases, the eruption was copious, but distinct, and the remaining cases assumed the form of varioloid, which in several amounted to little more than a mild eruptive fever. In five weeks, pratique was granted to all, no other cases having made their appearance in the other vessels of the squadron.

During the past summer, while the Ohio was in the harbor of Toulon, with a complement of more than nine hundred men, a case of small pox made its appearance in a man, who had not been on shore for some weeks. He was immediately removed to the civil hospital, on shore ; and here he recovered, after having had the disease severely. Strange to say, this was the only case which presented itself among this large number of men confined to the same ship. Small pox may be said always to prevail on the shores of the Mediterranean, but it is usually so mild as to require but little treatment. In Toulon, where it is almost at all times to be found in the fleet, quarantine is not enforced for this disease, while elsewhere, even in our own country, ships are not allowed pratique so long as it is found on board.

Extensive wound of the lung.—A young man from the Ohio, a servant of Lieutenant Ganzevoort, was admitted with a wound of the right lung from a blow with a Spanish knife. He was carrying a bundle in one of the most public parts of the town, when a Spanish soldier stole upon him from behind, and with one blow plunged a knife into the upper and posterior portion of the right lung. The weapon passed over the edge of the scapula, entering the thorax between the first and second ribs. He ran to the first door, holding on to his bundle, and fell senseless. We reached him soon after the receipt of the wound, and found him expectorating large quantities of blood, the internal hæmorrhage being very profuse, indicating that the large blood-vessels at the upper part of the lung had been divided. Our first object was to induce syncope, which was readily effected by opening the wound and allowing the blood to flow freely from it. The *deliquium animi* being complete, there followed for the time an arrest of the hæmorrhage, and we now contused the arterial branches within reach by torsion and compression. The intercostal artery was not divided, but judging from the copious hæmorrhage, the knife must have penetrated deep into the substance of the lung. The edges of the wound were brought into apposition by a deep interrupted suture, and the application of a compress and bandage. The patient was ordered to be kept perfectly quiet, and not even permitted to speak, and two grains of the acetate of lead were ordered every two hours, with directions to increase the quantity should there be a return of the hæmorrhage. The loss of blood had been very great, and the patient was almost completely exhausted in consequence of it; and this for the time was the only means by which the internal bleeding could be arrested. On the following morning he was found tranquil, not having had a return of the hæmorrhage. Upon auscultation, it was found that the function of the right lung, in consequence of the internal effusion of blood, had been almost entirely suspended, respiration being carried on by the lung of the opposite side. An enema was ordered, which had the desired effect; the acetate of lead was still continued, but at greater intervals; and cooling acidulated drinks were given in small quantities.

The following notes of the case were taken at the time:

Third day. There is some expectoration of blood during the night; he complains of pain and soreness in the right chest; but the external wound is healing by the first intention. Seidlitz powders ordered every two hours, until the bowels shall be moved, also an infusion of sem. lini, acidulated, for a common drink, with perfect rest.

It may be here remarked that, a short time prior to the admission of this case, our attention had been directed to an article in the Medico-Chirurgical Review, upon the advantages of high temperature after injuries and important surgical operations; and we determined to give this method of treatment a fair trial in this case of wounded lung, in which the influence of temperature might be supposed to be of much importance. The temperature of the apartment was consequently at all times kept as high as the patient could endure it without inconvenience, and in so doing we had no reference to the thermometer, which, for the three weeks immediately succeeding the accident, never fell below seventy degrees, and usually stood near seventy-six. To this high temperature we attribute, in a great degree, the recovery of this patient from a most formidable wound; and the efficacy of this treatment we have since had ample opportunity of testing in various cases. Indeed, no means with which we are acquainted promotes union so rapidly in lesions of all the tissues, including even fractures of the large bones, as a high temperature; and we should be happy were the favorable opinion here expressed to call the attention of the profession to its importance. The only point to be guarded against is never to carry the heated atmosphere to the extent of producing oppression or exciting the patient; and as the natural heat of the body, preserved by clothing, is not sufficient to effect the object in view, it must be done by the high temperature of the atmosphere which surrounds the patient.

Fifth day. The surface of the wound has completely united, but there is evidence of incipient emphysema; the subjacent parts are elevated and puffed, the lower costa of the scapula projects, and there is daily an expectoration of blood, which gradually diminishes in quantity. On the removal of the suture, the newly cicatrized wound opened readily, allowing a quantity of air and serum to make their escape. As the

4*

bowels are constipated, in consequence of the free use of the acetate of lead, ol. ricini ℥j. was ordered, which operated freely.

Seventh day. The patient is much more comfortable, which has been the case ever since the wound commenced discharging. There is a constant oozing of serum mixed with small bubbles of air; the tumefaction under the scapula is much reduced; the right side and shoulder are much discolored from ecchymosis; respiration has become more natural, and is unaccompanied with pain.

· Tenth day. This morning there is a slight return of hæmorrhage from the lungs; ordered the acetate of lead to be resumed, and an enema to be administered.

Fourteenth day. The discharge of serum and air from the wound has daily diminished in quantity; the respiration has become easy, the patient being now able to breathe in the horizontal position, having been heretofore obliged to remain with his chest almost erect; a more nutritious diet allowed.

Nineteenth day. The wound has again united; free expectoration; respiration is daily improving, in proportion to the absorption of the effused blood. Eight weeks after the receipt of the wound, the patient was returned to duty on board ship.

Recovery from gun-shot and even incised wounds of the lower lobe of the lungs is of frequent occurrence, but from such an injury of the upper lobe, death usually follows. The happy termination of this case, we must attribute to the syncope from the loss of blood, immediately after the injury was received, and perhaps to the beneficial effects of the high temperature preserved throughout the treatment.

It is scarcely necessary to add, that the soldier who perpetrated this outrage escaped, for these troops have been completely demoralized by the seven years civil war in Spain. Had the assassin even been arrested in the act, the governor, himself a soldier of fortune, would not have had sufficient firmness to punish him; for, should he have done so, his own life would have been forfeited to the troops by whom he was surrounded.

At the end of the last quarter for 1840, twenty-four patients were under treatment in the hospital. Of these, five were cases of injuries, nine of affections of the chest, and five of the stomach and bowels. Fifteen had been returned to duty cured, one died, and two were discharged the service at their own request.

From the first of January, 1841, until the thirteenth of March, twenty-seven were admitted, including eleven cases of psora in boys. Seven of the patients labored under pulmonary affections, two had disease of the intestinal canal, two had rheumatism, and three were cases of fractures. Two of the cases last mentioned are particularly worthy of notice.

Cases of Comminuted Fracture.—One of them, a marine, when intoxicated on shore, was knocked down by a party of Spanish soldiers, and while down, with his arms resting on the stone flagging, a large rock, weighing nearly one hundred pounds, was thrown upon his elbow, producing a comminuted fracture and a dislocation of the condyles of the humerus, both the ulna and radius being fractured. As his arm was large and muscular, the inflammation and swelling which immediately followed the injury, rendered it difficult to ascertain the precise situation of the comminuted fragments of the shattered bones; but these being adjusted as near as possible to their proper position, the injured joint was covered with leeches. After several days' rest, during which time the inflammation was reduced, it was determined, upon consultation with the surgeon of the fleet, that the limb should be kept extended, as that position brought the fractured olecranon and other fragments nearest their natural state. Although attempts were made to move the joint as soon as it could be done with safety, yet anchylosis could not be prevented.

The other case occurred in the person of a seaman, who had been on shore on liberty. Having been taken in charge by an officer, who was endeavoring to bring him on board, he threw himself over a precipice nearly forty feet in height, the officer himself narrowly escaping being carried with him. Fortunately he landed on a tiled roof beneath, which, giving way, broke the force of the fall, or he would doubtless have been instantly killed. He was conveyed to the hospital; and here, upon examination, it was discovered that the left tibia was fractured near the ancle-joint, and also two of the ribs on the right side, as well as the clavicle. The body generally was much bruised; and in addition to these ills, he was laboring under delirium tremens. The fractured leg was placed in Desault's apparatus, and tied down to the cot. Venesection ℥xvj. and tinct. opii et assafœtidæ were ordered. During the first twenty-four hours after his admission, he suffered greatly from delirium, and much force was necessary to prevent his moving the fractured bones; but after that, he became more tranquil, which was followed by a sound sleep; and thus we were enabled to direct our attention to a more perfect adjustment of the fractures. On the fourth day he was placed upon the fracture cot, which we invariably use in all cases of fracture of the lower extremities, both at sea and in hospital practice; but it is for the treatment of fractures on board ship that we were led first to construct it; and for this it is peculiarly adapted. Bandages and compress were applied to keep the ribs and clavicle in their proper position; and this was readily accomplished, as the patient was necessarily confined to the horizontal position. No apparatus can, indeed, so well adjust the fractured extremities of a broken clavicle as the method here pursued; and from this time, until the entire recovery of the patient, not a single unfavorable symptom was presented, notwithstanding the existence of four fractured bones, and the extensive injuries in other parts of the body.

Treatment of Fractures at Sea. This constitutes one of the most critical, as well as one of the most frequent duties of the naval surgeon; and almost every one who has had the treatment of such cases on board ship, has doubtless had the painful and disagreeable duty devolve upon him, to readjust the fracture,—an event that no care on his part or that of his patient can prevent. Not unfrequently, after the greatest vigilance and care, the naval surgeon has the mortification to find that the cure is not so perfect as it should be; and these *opprobria medicorum* of the naval surgeon are often brought up in judgment against him, by those who know but little of the countless difficulties encountered in the treatment of fractures at sea, especially in gales of wind, when those with sound limbs are unable to keep their feet, and the knees and timbers of the good ship herself are groaning and tearing asunder, as she sports about on the mighty waves. We have witnessed cases of deformity which had been treated by surgeons, whose eminence and reputation are a sufficient guarantee that everything had been done which judicious and careful attentions could effect toward preventing these unfortunate results. In a case, therefore, of so much difficulty, and one of such frequent occurrence, it is with no ordinary pleasure that we are enabled to recommend to the profession, as well as to all those " who go down upon the sea in ships," a fracture cot, which will effectually guard against all accidents from displacement. This apparatus, as represented in the lithograph facing the title-page, must, from its many advantages, and especially its simplicity, recommend itself to the profession. We are gratified in being able to add that such of our naval surgeons as have seen it in use, give it their highest approbation; and moreover, that it has met with the warm approval of several of the most experienced surgeons in the British and French service, by whom, when the apparatus was in use, it was carefully examined.

The apparatus consists of an ordinary ship's cot, eight feet long and three feet six inches wide, without sides. On the centre of this cot, the matrass and bedding of the ordinary size are to be made up, excepting the sheets and pillows; the head of the matrass is to be kept near to the head of the cot; and thus will be left a space of two feet between the lower end of the matrass and the foot of the cot. Over this, a large cot-frame or stretcher, also eight feet by three feet six inches, is to be suspended, by means of a tackle, as is seen in the plate. The canvas covering this frame is to have a hole, three feet and a half from its head, for the use of a bed pan; and on this frame the sheets and pillows are to be placed. Upon this moveable stretcher the patient remains throughout the treatment.

As this frame can be elevated or depressed at pleasure, every necessity can be attended to without the least motion on the part of the patient. The cot may be daily removed, aired, or changed, which is so frequently necessary in warm climates; and thus can cleanliness be more perfectly preserved than by any other method; while the fracture is at no time disturbed. When lowered down, the matrass beneath, upon which the patient rests, should always be within the frame of the stretcher; and this, by the way, is the only point necessary to guard against in the use of the cot; but its whole construction is so simple, that every forecastle-man will be able to make one.

Fractures at sea are displaced in consequence of the limb or splint coming in contact with the sides, or end of the cot, during the pitching or rolling of the ship, or in moving the patient while using the bed pan. This fracture cot, however, is without sides, and the end is never touched; a slight pull upon the tackle will elevate the patient without any effort on his own part, at the same time that the whole body moves together; and, whether he is resting in the cot upon the matrass, or is suspended over it upon the stretcher, he always moves free in space, with the motion of the ship, without any occasion for muscular exertion. Our limits will not permit our going farther into the merits of this invention, but its simplicity and usefulness will always be its best recommendation. Indeed, a fracture cot of this description should at all times be in readiness on board our ships of war, and on our excellent and incomparable European packets.

DESCRIPTION OF THE FRACTURE-COT.

aa Cot, eight feet long, and three feet six inches wide, without sides.
bb Matrass of the usual size—the head to be kept within six inches of the head of the cot, while a space of two feet is allowed below.
cc Life lines at the side of the cot.
dd A cot frame, or stretcher, covered with canvass, eight feet long, and three feet six inches wide, on which the sheet and pillows are to be placed.
e Hole for bed pan.
This frame is to be suspended over the cot, as seen in the plate, by a tackle; and during the treatment it is to rest upon the matrass, and is never to be raised except as occasion may require.

From the commencement of the quarter up to the 13th of March, twenty-four were returned on board ship, for duty. One had died, and two were discharged the service agreeably to their own request, leaving twenty-two under treatment on the day that we were detached from duty at the hospital, and ordered for service on board the United States' frigate Brandywine, Captain W. Compton Bolton.

During the time that the hospital was under our charge, the total number of admissions amounted to two hundred and nine. Of these, one hundred and forty-one were discharged cured, six were discharged at their own request, twenty-nine returned as invalids to the United States, and eleven died. Of the deaths, eight were from pulmonary affections,—a disease to which the records of the ships of the squadron are by no means favorable, notwithstanding the mildness of the climate and the reputed salubrity of the atmosphere of the Mediterranean. But it must be remembered, that the exposure to all weather on board ship, the wet decks, and the peculiar thoughtlessness of seamen, and perhaps their mode of life, would contribute to produce this disease to a much greater degree than in those who reside on shore. We are satisfied, however, that in no part of the world in which we have served, have we encountered so many cases of phthisis as among the Mahonese, —a result that admits of ready explanation in view of the endemic influence of the depressing passions, so universally excited into action through the governmental causes already detailed. Of the fatal cases at the hospital, the majority occurred in individuals who arrived on the station in comparative health, and in these, the progress of the disease was rapid. Among this number, were Assistant Surgeons Magil and Harrison, who, both educated at the University of Virginia, and both citizens of that State, were cut off by this disease at the very threshold of the most promising and useful career. One case of tracheal phthisis,—the purser of the Brandywine,—was much improved by the climate of the Mediterranean. Although his voice was at one time almost lost, accompanied with general atrophy, and, in a word, the presence of some of the most unfavorable symptoms; yet with care, and passing much of his time in Italy, the atmosphere of which is more genial, he improved far beyond the expectation of his friends, and returned to the United States almost completely restored. This case then affords positive evidence that, at least in Italy, the pul: monary invalid, even in cases apparently the worst, may reasonably expect some relief.

The number of cases treated in this hospital, bear but a small proportion to those of many other similar civil and military institutions; but upon examination, it will be found that the general character of the cases is totally different. While in hospital practice, generally, the mass of admissions present cases of an ordinary nature, here almost every case exhibited highly important features. These patients were all in apparent good health when joining their respective ships, and the cases had generally been under the care of able and experienced surgeons on board ship; and it was only in cases of an aggravated character, and often hopeless condition, that the patients were transferred on shore to enjoy the quiet and comforts which could not be obtained on board. Many cases possessed much interest from being the result of change of climate; and invalids arriving at the hospital presented opposite characters of disease, which do not occur in private practice. Two ships, arriving on the same day, one from the European shores, will have her invalids suffering from inflammatory affections and diseases of the respiratory organs; while the other, from the coast of Egypt or Syria, will have malignant dysentery and fever. In addition to these labors, the duties of the naval surgeon are materially augmented in consequence of the proverbially careless and reckless character of seamen. A majority of the cases which terminated fatally were in a hopeless condition at the time of reaching the hospital, and as all hopes of recovery were consequently idle, the efforts of the surgeon were limited to soothing their last moments,—to bestowing such attentions as we shall all ultimately require from each other, in the downward passage to the grave.

MEDICAL STATISTICS

OF THE

UNITED STATES FRIGATE POTOMAC,

COMMODORE JOHN DOWNES, COMMANDER,

DURING A THREE YEARS' VOYAGE CIRCUMNAVIGATING THE GLOBE.

THE United States Frigate Potomac, 44, bearing the pennant of Commodore John Downes, with a complement of five hundred men, performed a voyage of circumnavigation of the globe, during a cruise of three years. During this period she traversed ninety-seven degrees of latitude, that is, from 40° N. to 57° S., crossing the equator six times. A period of nearly two years was passed between the tropics; and it may be here added, as not a little singular, that while three months were spent within 6° of the equator in the East Indies, where a malignant dysentery made its appearance on board, the same period, subsequently, was passed in the same latitudes at the direct antipodes, in the vicinity of the Gallapagos Islands, where, from the absence, no doubt, of marshes, rank vegetation, and consequently of malaria, (notwithstanding these causes are not considered by many essential to the production of malarial diseases,) the crew enjoyed the average health of our own latitudes.

A concise statistical account of the health of the crew, with a brief notice of the character of the diseases developed in the different climates traversed, as well as those resulting from the confinement of so large a body of men on board ship, may not be uninteresting to the profession, as well as to the general inquirer. These, together with some brief observations upon the medical topography of the most important ports visited, are here presented from our notes and journal made during three years of active service and privations at sea, in the hope that they may prove interesting to some comfortably-seated fireside-traveller at home.

In entering upon the details of this voyage, we would bespeak the patient indulgence of the reader, confident that the general deductions, at least, will be interesting to the physician, the philanthropist, and the political economist.

We reported for duty on board the Potomac on the 22d of May, 1831, at which time two hundred and fourteen of her crew were on board. On the day of joining, twenty-four were upon the sick report, consisting of slight cases of indisposition usually encountered among new recruits. On the 3d of June, the ship hauled off from the navy-yard at Washington, to Greenleaf Point, (a distance of two miles,) into deep water; and here her armament and stores were received on board.   Throughout the day the crew, exposed to a very hot sun, labored hard and drank freely of the river water alongside.   During the night and the following day, many, in consequence, doubtless, to a great extent, of the impurities of the water drunk, were seized with cholera morbus, accompanied with violent spasms, which, in several robust young men, required copious venesection; but the disease readily yielded to treatment.   As the ship was immediately after watered and no more cases occurred, its relation with the river-water seems the more obvious.   The sick list was increased from twenty-two to thirty-six in one day, in consequence, no doubt, of this indulgence in the use of the river-water.

On the 15th of June we left Washington for Hampton Roads, where we arrived on the 22d.   The change from a fresh water river to the waters of the bay, materially improved the health of the crew, several cases of vernal intermittents having been speedily cured.   The sick list, for the number of men on board, continued large, having a daily average of twenty-three during the twenty-four days that we remained at Norfolk; and this high ratio was kept up by the new drafts of men, who came on board after the most violent debauchery and dissipation.   A very valuable seaman, who had been appointed boatswain, visited the shore on the 4th of July, to congratulate himself upon the receipt of his warrant; and after three days' absence, he was brought on board laboring under mania a potu and hæmoptysis, which proved fatal on the third day after his return.

On July 16th, we sailed for New York, with three hundred and fifty of the crew on board; and in five days we anchored off the battery, in the harbor of that city.   The full complement of the officers and crew having been here made up, and all the supplies furnished, the Potomac sailed, on the 24th of August, 1831, with five hundred and two souls on board.   All were in apparent good health, excepting one officer, affected with tracheal phthisis, whose case will be noticed in the sequel.   The average age of the crew, as near as could be ascertained, was thirty-one years.

In our passage toward the equator, we did not encounter the north-east trade winds, those of a variable kind and light airs having prevailed until we reached the third degree of north latitude; and here we met the south-east trades, which continued, with uniform regularity and force, until our arrival at Rio de Janeiro.   After passing the Cape de Verd islands, our course for eight days was parallel with the coast of Africa, distant four hundred miles; and here we encountered the most violent rains, accompanied with thunder and lightning, a high temperature, and thick, sultry, disagreeable weather.   Several cases of remitting fever presented themselves in these latitudes, but they did not assume a violent form.   On the 6th of October we crossed the equator; the thermometer was 79°, with fresh trade winds, and cloudy weather; and twenty-eight were on the sick report.   The passage from New York to Rio was made in fifty-three days; and during this time, the mean elevation of the thermometer at noon was 76°. Twelve cases of fever occurred, and ten were treated for injuries. Of the younger part of the crew, who had not been to sea previously, many suffered much from the confinement on board ship and the change of diet; and several obstinate cases of sea-sickness continued throughout the passage.

During our stay of twenty days in the harbor of Rio, the crew were freely supplied with fresh provisions, and were permitted to indulge without restraint in the delicious tropical fruits, which were very abundant. The mean of the thermometer at noon was 76°, that of the barometer 29.70 in., and the daily proportion on the sick report was seventeen.

The harbor of Rio is in 22°30′ south latitude, just within the tropic of Capricorn. It is equally unrivalled for its extent, its numerous deep bays, and its incomparable scenery ; and notwithstanding its intertropical location, it is exempt from malignant diseases, the yellow fever being there unknown. It also escaped the ravages of that dreadful scourge, the cholera epidemica. The inhabitants, however, far from enjoying vigorous health, are of a bilious temperament, feeble, and short-lived. Cutaneous diseases prevail to a great extent, and the streets are crowded with beggars suffering from leprosy and elephantiasis. Ships of war that remain a long period in this port usually have large sick lists, consisting, in a majority of cases, of diseases of the alimentary canal. Chronic diarrhœa is here very insidious in its invasion, and often terminates in incurable ulcerations. The rainy season is the most healthy, but ships' crews cannot be too carefully sheltered by awnings from the sun and rain ; and they should carefully abstain from the unripe fruit, which is brought off in great quantities by the bomb-boats.

Having sailed on the 5th of November for the Cape of Good Hope, we anchored in Table Bay on the 6th of December, after a passage of thirty-one days. The passage was boisterous, with much rain and thick foggy weather; the easting was made between the 32° and 34° of south latitude, strong westerly winds prevailing; and the thermometer averaged near 60° at noon throughout the passage. Forty were admitted with dysentery and diarrhœa on the passage ; and of these most occurred immediately after leaving port, and required treatment until our arrival at the Cape. The average number on the sick report during the passage, was twenty-one. The cold and wet weather induced a return of intermittent fever in twelve, who had had previous attacks ; but the disease readily yielded, after our reaching Table Bay, where intermittents are of rare occurrence.

The mean annual temperature at the Cape of Good Hope is about 68°, and the climate appears to be very favorable to health, in both natives and foreigners. Instances of longevity are numerous in the various races of men met with here, among whom are the Caffres, Hottentots, African Dutch-boors, and the English residents. The bills of mortality exhibit all the variety of disease to be met with in the same latitude north, while the violent and fatal diseases of warm climates are unknown. Invalids from British India often resort to this place for the restoration of health, many of whom, as we were informed, derive much benefit from the change.

In 1833, according to the British army statistics, the deaths were only six hundred and eighty-one out of a population of thirty-one thousand one hundred and sixty-seven, being one in forty-six, while in England according to the last census, the proportion was one in forty-seven and one-half. When it is considered that among the deaths at Cape Town, many were invalids who arrived there in the last stage of disease, and moreover that in some of the neighboring districts, the mortality for 1833 was only one in sixty-seven, which is a lower ratio than in the healthiest counties of England, it is obvious that, so far as regards the resident population, the climate is certainly not less favorable to the constitution than that of Britain. Among the British troops serving here, nearly two-thirds of the admissions into hospital are of that description which seldom prove fatal. Of the more serious diseases, the following is the order of their prevalence :—those of the stomach and bowels, those of the lungs, fevers, rheumatic affections. Intermittent and remittent fevers are extremely rare, they being, it is said, entirely unknown among the native inhabitants. In pulmonary affections, the climate is regarded as decidedly favorable.

Southeast winds prevail here, and frequently blow with great violence; and when this occurs, they are accompanied with a remarkable phenomenon, viz. : a small stationary cloud, which hangs over Table Bay, in the midst of the most violent tempest. Table Mountain and the white sandy beach of the bay, form the section of an amphitheatre, upon which an African sun glows with intense ardor; and from this heated surface, a highly rarified air ascends, until it attains the elevation of Table Mountain, when it comes in contact with the south-east winds, surcharged with humidity in their long passage over the Indian Ocean ; and as the dew-point is thus suddenly reached, the cloud in question is formed ; but, as it gradually attains the temperature of the surrounding atmosphere, the humidity is again absorbed, so that there is a constant generation and destruction, in the midst of a tempest, of this remarkable stationary cloud. While the Potomac remained, the mean temperature at noon was 78°.

On the 12th of December we sailed from Table Bay. Immediately after doubling the Cape we encountered a violent gale from the west; and a rough sea, and cold, wet weather, with westerly winds, continued until we made the island of St. Paul's. Several cases of pleuritis occurred, and many suffered from catarrh and rheumatism up to this period.

From the Island of St. Paul's, our course was northeast to Quallah-Battoo on the west coast of Sumatra, where this ship had been ordered to redress a piracy and murder, committed upon the ship Friendship of Boston. The crew were formed into division, and exercised whenever the weather would permit, in the use of fire-arms and the cutlass, to prepare them for the landing among these piratical and treacherous Malays; and such was the excitement upon the subject, and the anxiety of all to participate in the affair, that the sick report was smaller during the passage of fifty-one days, than at any other period of the cruise. The daily proportion sick was ten ; and upon our arrival at Quallah-Battoo, but three were unable to attend to duty, out of a crew of more than five hundred. The equator was crossed on the 27th of January, the thermometer being at 76°, with steady fresh south-east trade-winds ; and on the 5th of February, we anchored off Quallah-Battoo.

On the morning of the 6th, the attack was made upon the town, dismantling and destroying three forts, by which we had eleven wounded and two killed. In one of the wounded, the ball traversed the right lung, entering on the right of the sternum, at the sixth rib, and passed out under the scapula, having carried with it pieces of his belt, cloth jacket, and shirt. The hæmorrhage from the lungs was relieved by copious venesection on the spot where he fell. He continued to improve slowly; and after the foreign substances mentioned above were discharged by means of an abscess in the right side, he recovered with a collapse of the lung. Nearly all the wounds were severe, and several were dangerous; but from the comfortable quarters on the gun-deck of the frigate, and the uniform temperature of the atmosphere, they all recovered with unusual rapidity. We remained twelve days, during which time the thermometer stood at 85°, at meridian of each day, with alternate land and sea breezes. The severe exertions of the crew at the time of the attack on shore, and the necessary subsequent labor and exposure in watering the ship, after a long period of light duty, produced a material change in the health of the crew; and this was promoted by the absence of excitement which had for a time prevailed among all, and perhaps also by causes of a climatic nature. The sick list of three, in one month, increased to fifty-seven. Fifty-two cases of disease of the bowels and twelve of bilious fever, were treated within the month, notwithstanding fresh meat and vegetables were daily served to all hands, and every precaution was used to protect the men from the sun.

We have here a confirmation of an extraordinary fact, recorded in the "Statistical Report on the Sickness and Mortality of the Army of the United States," embracing the period from 1819 to 1839 :—

"It is, indeed, a remarkable fact in the medical history of fleets and armies, that, during the active progress of warlike operations, troops are little subject to the influence of disease. It seems as though the excitement of the passions has the power of steeling the system against the agency of morbific causes. On the contrary, as soon as the excitement is withdrawn, by a cessation of operations and a return to the monotony of a garrison, the constitution manifests the consequences of recent fatigue and exposure."

The Malays in this vicinity, which is in 4° north latitude, are healthy and robust, compared with their Asiatic and Javanese neighbors. They are very temperate in their habits, use but little animal food, and, like all Mahomedans, bathe frequently. Our numerous merchant vessels which have for years visited this coast, engaged in the pepper trade, enjoy comparative health, and apprehend but little danger when on the coast of Sumatra; while the shores of Java and Borneo, on the contrary, are shunned as we do a pest-house.

The topographical configuration of the west coast of Sumatra will readily account for its salubrity. Bold hills and spurs of mountains extend down to the sea; and although nature here revels in perpetual verdure, and there is a constant decay of vegetable matter, yet there are no fens and marshes, the mountain streams being precipitated with rapidity to the sea. Mount Ophir of Solomon is directly inland from this port, being distinctly visible whenever the atmosphere is free from clouds. We met with many of the natives who had suffered recently from small pox; and goitre was very common among them,—a disease which here at least cannot be attributed to snow-water as the exciting cause, for snow never falls even upon the mountains. On the 16th of February, we sailed from the west coast of Sumatra, and crossed the

5*

equator on the 20th, with the thermometer at 85°. On the 25th, the
sick list was again reduced to thirty, no new cases of diarrhœa having
been admitted since leaving port; and the wounded were all doing well.

On the 28th, we anchored in Bantam Bay, on the northwestern
extremity of Java, just within the Straits of Sunda. A change was
here made in the ration by order of Commodore Downes, which
contributed materially to the preservation of the health of the ship's
company. Portions of the beef, pork, and beans, which constitute the
navy ration, were discontinued, and rice and curry served out in lieu of
them. The spirit ration was divided into three portions, one of which
was given in the morning, one at noon, and the other in the evening.
All hands were ordered to wear flannel; and they were daily inspected
at quarters by the officers, to see that the order was complied with.
At Bantam Bay, we remained twelve days, wooding and watering
ship; and during this period, the mean temperature at noon was 82°,
with the regular land and sea-breezes, and several showers every day.
Fifteen cases of dysentery and four cases of fever, were admitted upon
the report, with a daily average of twenty-nine sick during our
stay.

On the 19th of March, we arrived at Batavia; and with a hope to
preserve the crew in good health, we anchored four miles from the
shore. This port has been more fatal to navigators than any other on
the globe. The largest and most valuable Indiamen have often here
been laid up for want of hands to navigate them, and here entire ships'
crews have found their graves. It was in this port that Dr. James
Johnson encountered the malignant fever which committed such
dreadful ravages in the English squadron in 1806, and which forms the
basis of his invaluable work upon the diseases of tropical climates. As
we were consequently not without the most dreadful forebodings, we
adopted every precautionary means of prevention that had heretofore
been found useful. Awnings were spread over the ship day and night,
—native Javanese boats' crews were employed to do the necessary
boat-duties of the ship,—the men were carefully sheltered from the
sun; in a word, all unnecessary duty was avoided. Those officers who
visited the shores, spent as little time as possible in the city. They
went directly into the country, where a purer atmosphere prevails, and
they strictly observed the most rigid temperance.

To Dr. Johnson we were much indebted for many valuable hints on
prevention; and after the occurrence of disease, we were enabled at
once to pursue a course of treatment, with the result of which we had
much occasion to be highly gratified. Indeed, to him we acknowledge
professional obligations, which it will ever be out of our power to
repay.

There was but little variation in the temperature during our stay at
Batavia, and the regular return of the land and sea breeze prevented
the heat from becoming oppressive; the mean at noon was 82°. When
the land breeze first reached us in the evening, it was charged with
the most offensive effluvia from the fens and marshes, which stretch
along the shores; and although anchored four miles from the land, this
noxious atmosphere was so oppressive, that all on board complained
much of it. This malaria doubtless brings with it the seeds of the
diseases from which strangers suffer so much.

The city is situated in 6° of south latitude, and is intersected by dykes

and canals, to which the Dutch settlers are so partial, and which materially contributed to its insalubrity. The walls which formerly
surrounded the town were removed, when in possession of Great
Britain, by Sir Stamford Raffles; and the city, at the same time, was
extended to the higher and more healthy grounds beyond, where at
present the foreign merchants and residents are congregated. The
governor and Dutch troops are stationed in the interior, where the
climate is less noxious to strangers; but a few years' residence in Java
is sure to be followed by physical and mental enervation.

Notwithstanding our precautions, the number of sick daily increased,
those reporting themselves sick suffering from a severe form of dysentery accompanied with much inflammation, tormina, and tenesmus.
In several cases, the disease assumed a most malignant character from
the commencement; and in one case, a robust, vigorous, young man,
it terminated fatally within twenty-four hours from the time of its
accession. Copious blood-letting, local and general, was ordered in
the commencement, and emetics administered to counteract the great
tendency to visceral congestion, and to restore a healthy action to the
deranged functions of the skin and liver. Mercurials in combination
with opium and ipecacuanha were regularly administered, and frequently with the most favorable results; and in conjunction with this,
mercurial inunctions were used, to accelerate the action of the mercury;
and when ptyalism occurred, the patient in almost every instance was
relieved, notwithstanding it did not in every case prevent a fatal termination. When this course of treatment did not arrest the progress
of the disease within a few days, bloody fœtid evacuations followed,
with gangrene, collapse, and death.

On the 10th of April, in consequence of the increase of sickness, we
sailed from Batavia with forty-two cases of dysentery on board. On
the 20th, we crossed the equator, the thermometer being at 90°, and
the sick report increasing. On the 21st, at meridian, at anchor one mile
north of the equator, the weather calm, and the thermometer at 85°,
fifty cases of dysentery were on the report, and new cases occurring
daily. Chloride of lime was used freely about the cots and hammocks
of the sick, and every possible attention was paid to cleanliness. On
the 1st of May, three deaths occurred within the preceding twenty-four
hours; but the number of cases was reduced to thirty-four, and no new
ones had appeared within several days. Since leaving port the thermometer averaged 84°, with calm and light airs. After being at sea
twenty days, we had sailed but six hundred miles, with a vertical sun,
being, indeed, almost directly under the equator. On the previous
night, we experienced the most tremendous thunder, lightning, and rain,
without wind; and on the following morning, we had a light breeze
which continued until our arrival at Canton, after a passage of thirty-
nine days. From this time, the health of the crew continued to improve.
One hundred and fifty cases of dysentery were registered within a few
weeks, among which there occurred but thirteen deaths,—a proportion
truly small, when compared with the number of fatal cases on board
other ships in the China seas.

The Potomac remained at the Island of Lintin for nineteen days;
the mean temperature at noon was 80°, with a fresh sea breeze which
thoroughly ventilated the ship. The average number on the sick report
was twenty-six, three-fourths of whom had chronic dysentery, and six

suffered from bilious fever. The Lintin fleet, which remains at anchor
here for many months at a time, usually enjoys good health; but
dysentery and fever, during some seasons, prove very fatal. Although
the native Chinese appear to suffer but little from the epidemic
diseases, yet they are but a feeble and enervated race. We were
informed by a resident American surgeon, that he had frequently met
with cases among the natives, in which fractures would not unite; and
ulcerations are also extremely difficult to heal, in consequence of this
debilitated state of the vital powers.

Ships going to the East Indies cannot be too careful in enforcing the
regulations adopted on board the Potomac; for, we were thereby
enabled to carry a larger number of men in safety through those seas,
than had probably ever before been accomplished. The less animal
food consumed, the better; and the entire abolition of the spirituous
portion of the ration, would, we are satisfied, be also attended with
much benefit in these excessively hot climes.

We sailed for the Sandwich Islands on the 5th of June, with thick
heavy weather, and a fresh breeze. On the ninth, during a typhon,
with the thermometer at 80°, there were two deaths from chronic
dysentery. The easting was made between the 34th and 36th degrees of
north latitude, with strong westerly winds and cool wet weather, which
completely changed the character of the diseases on board. Pleuritis,
intermittents, and inflammatory affections, took the place of dysentery;
but they were not of an aggravated character. Twenty-five was the
average on the sick report for the passage.

We arrived at Oahu, Sandwich Islands, on the 23d July, after a passage
of forty-eight days; and here we remained for twenty-three days. During
this period, the mean of the thermometer at noon was at 78°, and
that of the barometer 29.90 in. The crew were here granted liberty—" a
run on shore,"—which was much enjoyed; and it was followed by a much
smaller increase in the number of sick, than generally ensues from
liberty in a port which has greater facilities for dissipation and intemperance. On the day of entering the port, seventeen were under
medical treatment, and at the time of sailing, twenty-two, which is a
very small number in view of the largeness of the crew.

The Sandwich Islands are situated in 20° north latitude. The
climate appears peculiarly favorable to the human constitution; for the
natives are extremely large and corpulent, and such as are accustomed
to labor, are possessed of great strength. This tendency to corpulency is
much encouraged, particularly in females, in whom it is considered the
greatest evidence of beauty; and to this result, their native food, the
aurum maculatum, or wake robin, is said to contribute in an especial
manner. This plant, which is cultivated with care, contains a large
portion of fecula, from which they manufacture starch, made into *poye*,
which, eaten with *raw fish*, is considered one of their greatest luxuries.
The natives suffer much from a species of leprosy, which they call the
craw-craws; and to cure which, they undergo a course of treatment
with the *kavaroot*,—a powerful alterative and narcotic. Upon the
arrival of the missionaries, infanticide was of very frequent occurrence.
To effect this purpose, they used a drastic, purgative, indigenous bean,
which not unfrequently destroyed the mother, and seldom failed to
produce abortion; but this horrid practice, through the salutary influence
of the missionaries, has been in a great measure discontinued.

We sailed for the Society Islands on the 15th of August, and crossed the equator on the 5th of September, in 5° west longitude, with the thermometer at 80°, and the south-east trades. At this time there were twenty-four on the sick report. Twelve cases of intermittent fever were admitted during the passage; and many of those laboring under dysentery continued to suffer upon our approach to the equator, from chronic diarrhœa. A few degrees north of the equator we met with calms and heavy rains, with the thermometer ranging above 80°, when these cases of relapse occurred. On the twenty-eighth day we anchored at the Island of Otaheite, having an average of twenty-seven under treatment for the time at sea. At this island the crew were much on shore, wooding and watering ship, the tropical fruits were procured in the greatest abundance, and no unpleasant consequences resulted from their use. We lost one of the crew while in this port, from concealed strangulated hernia. This island, which is in latitude 16° south, consists in its interior of high volcanic mountain land, surrounded by a fertile belt of rich alluvial deposit near the shores. The climate is truly delightful, and all the wants of the natives are supplied by the spontaneous productions of nature. The natives have not so great a stature as those of the Sandwich Islands; but they are more gay and cheerful in their character, and many of the females are delicate and graceful. A light complexion is much esteemed among them, to improve which they avoid the sun, and bathe themselves with the juice of the *papa*, which is an indigenous plant. Their diet consists of fresh vegetables, fruit, and fish, of which the bread-fruit constitutes the principal; and as all the tropical fruits are here produced spontaneously, labor is unnecessary, and their lives are consequently inactive and indolent. The Missionaries who remain some time in the Society Islands, seldom escape an attack of elephantiasis. We met with two who suffered from this disease in a most aggravated form. The natives also suffer much from this affliction.

The passage between Otaheite and Valparaiso in Chili was made in the vicinity of the thirty-fifth degree of south latitude; and as it was in the winter of the southern hemisphere, much colder weather was encountered than we had previously met with, accompanied with rain, wind, and a rough sea. The ship was exceedingly uncomfortable, and the change of weather once more completely revolutionized the type of disease. Fifteen cases of pneumonia and pleuritis, with twenty-two cases of rheumatism, were admitted upon the sick report. Milder forms of catarrh and inflamed tonsils were numerous, and the general liability of the crew to indisposition, upon exposure and bad weather, indicated that all began 'to suffer from the long period passed at sea. After a passage of thirty-four days, we arrived at Valparaiso, having had an average of thirty-six patients, who required careful treatment during the voyage. Besides, many had been excused from duty, from time to time, in consequence of slight indisposition, but who were not placed on the sick report. Among the number sick on this passage were two cases of scurvy, which did not manifest themselves until we came under the influence of the land air. The first few days in port aggravated the disease, but as the symptoms were mild, the patients speedily recovered; and these were the only cases of scurvy which presented themselves during the cruise. The Potomac arrived at Valparaiso, which is in the same longitude with New York, on the twenty-fourth of October, 1832, having been fourteen months from the United States, nearly twelve of which had been passed at sea.

Soon after arriving, liberty was given to the crew, which, as usual, for a few days, more than doubled the number on the sick report. Eleven were treated for mania a potu, and many contracted syphilis. We remained forty days in port, during which time the crew were freely supplied with fresh provisions, and were allowed relaxation after a long period of active service at sea. The mean of the thermometer at noon was 66° and that of the barometer 29.75 in. This is here the season of spring; high winds prevail from the south, without rain. The number sick averaged nearly forty for each day in port, a majority of them suffering from the effects of the cruise on shore, and the consequent dissipation.

Valparaiso, which is in 33° south latitude, is surrounded by spurs of the Andes, which run down in bold bluffs to the sea. The climate is one of the most salubrious in the world; and to the early Spanish conquerors, who reached it after their invasion of Mexico and Peru, where they suffered much from the intense heat and arid soil, this port was so enchanting that it received the name of the "vale of Paradise." Santiago, the capital of Chili, is ninety miles inland, at the foot of the Cordillera, with a population of nearly fifty thousand. The capital is remarkable for sudden vicissitudes of temperature, the days being very hot, while the nights are cold. This is occasioned by the snow-clad mountains near the city, the cold atmosphere from their summits descending into the highly rarefied atmosphere of the plains below. Remittent and intermittent fevers are very common, as well as rheumatism, and the whole class of phlegmasiæ, which invariably result from extremes of heat and cold. Goitre is frequently met with, every individual in some families being affected with it,—a disease which the natives, as in Switzerland, attribute to the use of the snow-water from the mountains, which supplies the town; but this explanation would surely be laughed at by the patients affected similarly, that we saw in the island of Sumatra. The various preparations of iodine have been found very efficacious in its treatment. While at Santiago we heard of a case of extirpation of the thyroid gland, which resulted in the death of the patient.

On the second of December we sailed for Lima, with the usual south wind, and arrived at Callao on the fifteenth, the sick report having been reduced to eighteen. We remained in this port for seventy-five days, during which period the ship's hold was broken out, and every part thoroughly cleaned and painted. The weather was uniformly clear, with a most delightful south wind; here it never rains, and at this season, mists and fogs are equally unknown; the mean of the thermometer at noon was 70°, and that of the barometer 29.85 in., with a daily proportion of twenty-four upon the sick report. Four cases of remitting fever were treated; there was but little arterial excitement, with much disturbance of the nervous system, and it was found that they would not bear the use of the lancet.

The city of Lima, which is in 12° south latitude, is eight miles from the bay. The inhabitants, although much enervated by the continued high temperature, and their dissipated and indolent lives, leading to premature old age, yet enjoy good, if not robust, health. Although foreigners suffer less from acute diseases than in India, yet they are insidiously worn down by the climate, notwithstanding the most extreme temperance and regularity in living. The streets of Lima are kept very clean, many having streams of water running through them; and to this must be added, as an additional cause of their exemption from malignant disease, the remarkable property of the atmosphere in producing dry putrefaction, which thus prevents all noxious effluvia. Dead animals are suffered to remain in the roads; and the Pantheon, in which all the dead of the city are interred, notwithstanding open to the air, never emits the least disagreeable effluvia. This property of the atmosphere arises from the large quantity of nitrate of soda diffused through it, from the soil, and which in situations that have not been disturbed for a long period, may be found deposited in small crystals. The long chain of the Andes, which forms the immense barrier along the entire western coast of South America, with an elevation of from twelve to eighteen thousand feet, completely interrupts the progress of the winds from the east, the only direction from which they blow along the coast of Peru, being from the south ; and as these south winds are much colder than the air they encounter in their progress towards the equator, and as their capacity for humidity consequently continues to increase, it follows that rain cannot form. Rain is consequently unknown in these countries; but as the winds reach the Isthmus of Darien, the air becomes surcharged with moisture, which is there precipitated in torrents.

Our ships of war pass much time in this port, with generally a large sick report. Dysentery sometimes prevails to a great extent, and during the months of July and August, when fogs prevail, those predisposed to tubercular phthisis are liable to have the disease developed. We here lost one of the crew from consumption; and an officer from the U. S. Ship Falmouth, who was seized with hæmoptysis, was transferred to the Potomac, in the hope that a change to Valparaiso would be of service; but the case terminated fatally soon after our return to Chili.

On the twenty-eighth of February, 1833, we sailed for Valparaiso, which we reached in sixteen days, after a cold, wet, and boisterous passage ; the mean of the thermometer was 64°, and the average number on the sick list was twenty-three. We remained in port sixty-seven days, during the months of March, April, and May, (these being the autumn months in Chili), with much colder weather than at the time of our previous visit. In May we had two severe northers, which, as the harbor is open to the north, are dangerous; and both were accompanied with rain. These northers, which are always indicated by the barometer, only occur at this season. The average on the sick report during our stay, was twenty-one; and this number was kept up in consequence of the liberty given to the crew on shore. Several cases of pleuritis, rheumatism, and inguinal adenitis, occurred in consequence of the exposure and the wet ship. At Lima, cases of chronic diarrhœa presented themselves, which were relieved soon after a change to a cooler climate.

On the twenty-fifth of April, a case of small-pox occurred in one of the servants, who contracted the disease on shore. As soon as the character of the affection was ascertained, the patient was transferred to an hospital on shore, to prevent its extension. Within a few days, another case made its appearance, and this was followed by a third, all of whom were sent on shore. On the first of May, during a norther, the thermometer fell to 40°, there being now a large sick list, composed chiefly of inflammatory affections. During our stay, fourteen were upon the report with scrofulous affections, twenty-two with pulmonary and hepatic inflammation, and sixteen with rheumatism. Four weeks having elapsed since the appearance of the last case of variola, it was thought that the disease had disappeared, and we consequently, on the twenty-second of May, sailed for Coquimbo, which we reached in three days; but on the eleventh of June other cases of variola presented themselves, which placed beyond a doubt the fact that the contagion was on board ship, and that it would inevitably extend throughout the entire ship's company. It was now determined to inoculate the whole ship's company, as we would thereby materially diminish the severity of the disease, and accelerate its progress throughout the ship; for, as long as it continued on board, we were subject to a most irksome quarantine. On the twentieth, all hands were called to muster; and beginning with the officers, every individual who was not marked with the small-pox was inoculated with lymph taken from a well-developed case on board. The number inoculated was two hundred and eighty-seven, all of whom had their grog stopped, and were daily furnished with fresh provisions. At this time the general health of the crew was very good, having an average of but eighteen on the report, exclusive of those suffering from small-pox.

Eighty-five of those inoculated took the disease, many of them having it in a very mild form. When there was a tendency to inflammation, or the febrile action ran high, venesection was ordered with small and repeated doses of the sulphas magnesiæ. The solution of supertart. potassæ was given as a common drink, and a low diet prescribed. In eleven cases, the eruption extended over the body; but in no case did it become confluent, nor was it accompanied by any unfavorable symptoms. The febrile excitement was most severe on the eleventh day after inoculation, from which time it gradually subsided. Thirteen of the crew were without any evidence of previous vaccination, all of whom took the disease from inoculation; and the eighty-five who became effected in this way, were consequently all susceptible to its influence.

While here in quarantine from small-pox, the American whale-ship "Corinthian," entered the port with this disease on board. There were three cases, two of which terminated fatally soon after her arrival. The remainder, twenty-seven, we inoculated, eleven of whom took the infection and recovered in proper time, without any unfavorable event. Of the three who took the disease in the natural way, two died, while eleven with the disease by inoculation, all recovered,—a result which presents strong testimony in favor of inoculation.

Coquimbo is very healthy, and it has a remarkable uniformity of temperature throughout the year. The city, eight miles from the landing, was called, by the old Spaniards, from the serenity of its atmosphere, La Serena, and it was selected, for the same reason, by the proprietors of the silver and copper mines, as their residence. To this purity of the atmosphere and uniformity of temperature, together with the careful inoculation of all on board, may be attributed the good fortune of not losing a man out of so large a crew, from this terrible disease. The average on the report, exclusive of the cases of variola, was nineteen; the thermometer averaged 69°, and the barometer 29.80 in. There had been no rain at Coquimbo for three years previous to our arrival, but while there we had several showers.

The cases of small-pox had so far improved by the eighth of July, that the Commodore was enabled to put to sea, with the usual south wind, which in eight days carried us to Callao. On the twenty-second of August we sailed from Callao, having passed thirty-five days in port; and during this time, the thermometer at noon averaged 71°, the barometer 29.77 in., and the daily ratio of the crew under medical treatment was twenty-eight.

This period is here the midst of the season of fogs and mist, when the atmosphere is continually obscured; and now is the time when the prevailing diseases of dysentery, fevers, and pulmonary affections, are rife. Several of the crew were down with remitting fever, which was insidious in its approach, accompanied with great prostration and a small and frequent pulse. Dr. Ruschenberger, the surgeon of the Falmouth, who had seen much of this disease on this coast, found the best treatment to consist in mild saline diaphoreties and regimen. Many of the crew suffered from an enlargement of the inguinal glands, which appears peculiar to the coast of South America, and in which suppuration, notwithstanding every care and attention, will follow. These cases of adenitis are unconnected with syphilis, and are extremely difficult of treatment on board ship. In three days we anchored at Payta; and here, although so short a distance from Callao, where we had recently been enveloped in fogs and mists, we found the atmosphere perfectly serene, with but little difference in the thermometer between day and night.

After a short stay, we sailed for the Gallapagos Islands; and on the first of September we anchored in Essex Bay, Charles Island, 1° 13' south latitude. This entire group of islands is of recent volcanic origin, one or more cones of craters being found on every one; and as regards soil, little has as yet accumulated to sustain the scanty vegetation. Until recently these islands have been uninhabited, the one at which we were anchored having a few people. The crew were much on shore, collecting the immense terrapins, for which these islands are celebrated; and notwithstanding the great labor of carrying these large animals over the broken lava, under a vertical sun, they remained in good health. It was in this port that Commodore Porter recruited his men, and procured fresh provisions during his cruise in the Essex in the last war. American whale-ships resort much to these islands for the same purpose, an additional inducement being found in the circumstance that the sailors are here unable to procure ardent spirits, and there is no danger of desertion. During the ten days that we remained in port, the mean of the thermometer was 73°, that of the barometer 29.90 in., and the average on the sick report, including several cases of dysentery, was twenty-one. All those here attacked with dysentery, had suffered from the same disease when at Batavia, the antipodes from our present position.

From the Gallapagos Islands we proceeded to Guayaquil, anchoring on the eighth day, at Puna, at the mouth of the river, in 2° south latitude. The crew were much predisposed to disease of the intestinal canal, particularly those who had previously suffered in the East. The number of cases of dysentery continued to increase, with acute inflammatory symptoms, tormina and bloody evacuations; but the disease did not assume that malignant type, nor was it so difficult of treatment as that of Batavia. Among thirty-eight cases of dysentery

6

and diarrhœa treated since our arrival in the vicinity of the equator, but two terminated fatally. Within the month, when in the same latitudes, eight cases of chronic hepatitis came upon the sick report, which yielded to mercurial alteratives, and the nitro-muriatic acid administered internally and by baths. While at Puna, the average on the report was thirty-two, a majority of whom were seriously unwell, and required much careful attention. Guayaquil is at all times very unhealthy, particularly during the rainy season, which continues several months. The quantity of rain that falls is very great; but as we could not ascertain that any rain-gauge had been kept, we are unable to give the quantity.

On the 28th of September we sailed for Payta, which was reached in three days, having now twenty-eight upon the sick report. A few days in this truly delightful atmosphere again reduced the number of sick to fifteen, which consisted of the convalescents with dysentery and diarrhœa. The climate of this port is one of the most salubrious on the coast of Peru, it being remarkable for uniformity of temperature, dryness of the atmosphere, and the regularity of the winds. The mean annual temperature is about 72°, and the mean of the barometer is 29.90 in.; and here the dense fogs of Lima, and the heavy rains of Guayaquil, are equally unknown. Payta is the port of Piura, a city with a population of four thousand, twenty miles inland on the Colon river. This river passes through marshes filled with the *sarsaparilla*, from which the waters are imputed to imbibe medicinal virtues, which, together with the salubrity of the atmosphere, makes this place the resort of invalids from the neighboring country. The sarsaparilla forms an important article of exportation.

The cruising grounds for the American ships employed in the sperm whale fisheries are directly off this port; and they frequently resort here for supplies, particularly for fruits and vegetables, as antiscorbutics, for which, in their long cruises, they are much in need. At the head of the list of antiscorbutics, among the whalers, stand raw potatoes; two are served out daily to each man, and eaten raw with vinegar, which, after a long confinement to salt provisions, are much relished by all hands. Those only who have been much at sea can know the longings for, and the luxury of, fresh vegetables of any description.

October 10th, we sailed for Lambayeque, where we touched on the 16th, and proceeded thence to Callao, which we reached on the 27th of the month. In our progress south the thermometer fell, and we again encountered the fogs and mists, which, for a time, we had left behind. At the period of our arrival, the sick report was increased to forty, the mean of the thermometer at noon, for the passage, being 62°. We remained twenty-seven days at Callao, the thermometer having a mean of 69°, and the barometer of 29.65 in., with an average of thirty upon the sick report, including several cases of scrofulous glandular affections, which are here found to be very obstinate.

On the 21st of November, we sailed from Callao, having at different periods of the cruise, spent one hundred and twenty-seven days in this port. The average number under treatment was larger here than at Valparaiso, consisting of cases of disease of the intestinal canal, and the obstinate cases of adenitis to which we have already alluded. In a few cases, where constant rest could be maintained, the use of the pediluvium and evaporating lotions, would effect a resolution; but these cases were rare; suppuration usually ensued, when for weeks and months we had to contend with indolent ulcers. The average number sick in this port during our visits at various seasons, was thirty-two.

The Limaians, the descendants of the Spanish conquerors, are rapidly decreasing, and promise, in their continued revolutions, soon to become extinct. They have uniformly lived in great luxury, as the proprietors of the valuable gold and silver mines; and for generations, they have been devoted to gambling and dissipation, which have rendered the present race short-lived and feeble. They are diminutive in stature, slight in form, and many of the females, when young, are exceedingly beautiful; but from the premature development of a warm climate,—a law which recent investigations show to have been much exaggerated,—they often become mothers at an early period, and consequently rapidly decline into premature old age. The native Peruvians, who at this time constitute seven-eighths of the population of the country, are short, with very large chests, and broad Chinese features; they are fond of agricultural pursuits; and as they were originally conquered by a mere handful of Spaniards, they still permit themselves to be governed by the same.

We would here respectfully, as a traveller, insert our protest against the declaration of our learned and distinguished countryman, Dr. S. G. Morton, who, in his elaborate volume upon the Crania of America, speaks thus:—"The concurrent testimony of all travellers goes to prove, that the native Americans are possessed of certain physical traits that serve to identify them in all localities, the most remote from each other, nor do they, as a general rule, assimilate less in their moral character and usages." In craniological formation, as well as in his moral character and usages, the Peruvian differs widely from his warlike and intellectual neighbor of North America. The physiognomy is entirely different, possessing but little intelligence, and being totally devoid of the noble intellectual expression of our northern Indians. Temple, who passed years among them, says that they resemble the Tartar or Chinese; and Burrow, who has written so ably upon their country, expresses his conviction of their descent from the Chinese; and as regards the native Mexicans, many of the most accurate observers, —as for instance, in the recent able work of Madame Calderon de la Barca,—advance the same opinion respecting their origin. Between this nation and the Peruvian, there is a close approximation in physical formation; and as regards habits and character, they are found precisely to correspond. The phrenological organization of the native Peruvian indicates but little intellectual development, while at the same time their animal propensities are also diminutive; and these indications are strongly corroborated by their habits and character. When left to themselves, unlike our northern Indians, they diligently cultivate their fields, live amicably with each other, and are hospitable and friendly. The striking analogy among the four hundred dialects of America, it is true, strongly confirms the opinion of a common origin, pertaining to all the American tribes; and all the differences found to obtain among them, may possibly be due entirely to the agency of climate and other causes. But these differences, physical, moral, and intellectual, are certainly much more strongly marked than the language of Morton, just quoted, would at all justify.

We arrived at Valparaiso in twenty-five days, having encountered calms and adverse winds, with an average of twenty-six under

treatment, for the passage. Off the island of Juan Fernandez we
encountered a gale, with the thermometer at 50°, which brought on
several cases of pneumonia and pleuritis. Six cases of hepatitis were
treated at sea; and as we approached the coast, the cold air from the
snow-clad Andes brought on catarrhs and colds, from which few escaped.
A few days in port restored the crew to health, as the weather at this
season is dry and temperate.

We remained fifty-three days in Valparaiso, with an average of
eighteen on the sick list, a majority being cases of slight injuries; but
there were several cases of bilious fever, which did not, however,
present any important features. A quarter gunner, one of the most
athletic and valuable men in the ship, lost his life from a fall on shore,
causing a fracture of one of the lumber vertebræ, and one case of phthisis
pulmonalis terminated fatally.

At this season, (the summer,) dysentery and fevers prevail among the
natives on shore, and acute cases of hepatitis also manifest themselves
during the warm weather. We were called in consultation in a case of
hepatitis in a Mr. Blanco, a gentleman who, educated at West Point,
promised much usefulness in this new country; but several previous
attacks had much enfeebled him, and suppuration taking place in
the liver, he died within a short time after our first visit. The total
number of days passed at Valparaiso at our different visits was one
hundred and sixty, with a uniformly small sick list, notwithstanding the
crew were allowed to go on shore frequently during each visit,—an
immunity from disease which must be due to their incomparable
climate.

The native Chilanoes are a robust and vigorous race, frequently
attaining a great age. Accustomed from youth to the open air, with
much active exercise, particularly on horseback, they are capable of
enduring great fatigue; and nowhere are men met with, who are
possessed of more iron constitutions than the inhabitants of these
mountains. An inflammatory fever prevails during the autumn, in the
interior, attended with much cerebral congestion, which sometimes
assumes the form of a fatal epidemic. By the natives it is thought to be
contagious, who give it the name of *chavolungo,* for which they administer
an infusion of an indigenous plant, the *conchelagua,* a powerful
diaphoretic. The condition of the medical profession, in both Chili
and Peru, is very low, there being no schools of medicine. The native
practitioners are from the lower orders of life, ignorant and uneducated,
and commanding but little respect. In the large cities, a few foreign
medical men are to be found, but their practice is limited to foreigners
and a few of the most affluent of the natives, the prejudices of the
lower classes being much against them.

On the 9th of February, we sailed for the United States; and we
encountered head winds until we reached the fiftieth degree of south
latitude, the thermometer falling as we advanced south, with much rain.
On the 6th of March we were off Cape Horn, in 57° south, with the
thermometer at 44°, and the barometer at 29.80 in., and thirty-six being
upon the sick report. The character of the diseases on board had
entirely changed since our departure from Valparaiso. Cases of
pleuritis, cynanche tonsilaris, and rheumatism, augmented the sick
report; and very many of the crew were very unwell, but unwilling to
go upon the sick list, as long as they were able to keep about on our

passage home. After doubling Cape Horn, fresh and favorable winds continued until our arrival at Rio de Janeiro, on the twenty-third of March. The average on the report of sick for the passage, was thirty-three, three-fourths of whom suffered from inflammatory affections, produced by the cold weather off the cape ; and a proportion daily of as many more were prescribed for, who still continued to perform their duty.

We remained sixteen days in Rio. Although this was the rainy season, with frequent showers during the day, yet the quantity of rain which fell was very small. The mean of the thermometer was 78°, that of the barometer 29.78 in., with twenty-one on the sick report.

After leaving Rio, a number of cases of diarrhæa were admitted for treatment, being no doubt the result of the heat and rain to which the men had been exposed in watering ship and bringing off the supplies. On the 27th of April we crossed the equator with the thermometer at 82°, with southeast trades, and twenty-seven on the sick report. We reached Boston on the twenty-third of May, after a passage of forty-four days, having had a daily average of twenty-eight sick. Upon our arrival in the United States, the health of the crew was such as to enable all but six to take their discharge. Of these, two had phthisis, one, a fracture of the leg, and the remaining three, chronic rheumatism ; all of whom were transferred to the naval hospital.

Having thus concluded the statistical details of this voyage, which, it is to be feared, have proved somewhat tedious, the deductions that follow cannot, however, but be regarded as of the highest interest and importance.

The Potomac had been in commission for more than three years, during which period the total number of deaths had been twenty-five, viz :

Dysentery,	16
Phthisis,	3
Hepatitis,	1
Concealed Hernia,	1
Hydrocephalus,	1
Fractured vertebræ,	1
Shot at Quallah Battoo,	2
Total,	25

Seven of the ship's company, including two of the junior officers, had been returned to the United States as invalids.

The average number of souls on board for three years was four hundred and ninety, including thirty commissioned and warrant officers. The annual ratio of deaths was therefore 2.08 per cent., which is much less than in the same number of adults on shore. It should be remembered, however, that at the time of sailing we were all in excellent health. The daily average of the number on the sick report for three years, was twenty-eight, which is surely a very small number out of a crew of five hundred, who had gone through the East Indies, and crossed the equator six times. Moreover, this was the first cruise of this ship, when, in consequence of the large quantities of salt used in their construction for the preservation of the timber, crews often suffer much from the humidity occasioned by the salt, which does not exist in her subsequent service. The United States Frigate Brandywine was very sickly on her first two cruises, which was attributed to her being freely salted,—an inference strengthened by the fact that since then her crews have enjoyed good health.

This frigate, as an experiment in our marine, had her galley on the berth-deck, where it was thought the heat from the fires would assist in the ventilation of the ship, at the same time that she would be kept dry between decks. There were unquestionably constant currents of air down the hatches and windsails toward the fire, at the same time that the highly rarefied air from below ascended; but this was more than counteracted by the suffocating heat of the large fires on the confined and crowded berth-deck, while the water constantly and necessarily in use in cooking, kept the lower deck wet. Besides, when the galley is placed there, cleanliness cannot be so well preserved, as when it is on the upper deck.

During the voyage of circumnavigation, the Potomac sailed over sixty-one thousand miles, having been at sea five hundred and fourteen days. She crossed the equator six times, varying from 40° north, to 57° south latitude; and in all this service, she had not a spar carried away, nor did she lose a man by any accident on board,—the strongest testimony of the excellent state of discipline, and the prudence and precaution of her commander.

In the cheerful and contented condition of the crew, with constant employment, can be traced the health of the whole ship's company; and to this end, theatrical entertainments, a weekly newspaper when at sea, and a relaxation from the severe military discipline during the long passage across the Indian and Pacific Oceans, as well as the judicious medical police enforced on board while in the most insalubrious ports on the globe,—all materially contributed. About one-third of the crew had the spirituous portion of the ration stopped for the cruise; but as that number embraced the boys and landsmen, who had never been at sea, they were more frequently on the sick list than the old seamen who drank their grog. The recent reduction in the quantity of grog, as well as the change in the ration, is probably the most important step yet taken toward the reformation and improvement of the character of the seamen and of the whole navy.

When we compare the health of the crew of the Potomac with that of early circumnavigators, the increased health of ships' companies at sea will be found truly surprising. Lord Anson sailed from England with eight vessels and one thousand nine hundred and eighty souls; and out of these, only a single ship's company, the Centurion, performed her voyage of circumnavigation. The early Spanish and Dutch navigators were equally unfortunate, and whole crews perished from the scurvy, —a disease which has been almost exterminated in modern days.

The great improvements in marine police, first adopted by Captain Cook during his voyages of discovery, among which was the introduction of the hammock for all on board, have benefited navigators as much as his geographical discoveries; but his vessels were small, which are always more healthy than large ones; his crews, at the same time, were in a constant state of excitement, anxiously looking forward toward the discoveries which they were constantly making; and they were also satisfied that they would receive a handsome reward and a warm reception, upon their return home. These precautions, in conjunction with cheerfulness and cleanliness, constitute the only good prophylactics on board ship.

One word more in regard to scorbutus. This horrible disease may be said to have been the universal scourge of the sea until the year 1795, when the British admiralty issued an order for furnishing the navy with a regular supply of lemon-juice, from which time the extinction of this horrid disease in that arm of the service may be dated. The destructive ravages of this disorder are awfully portrayed in the narratives of the early English navigators, particularly in those of Sir Francis Drake, Davis, and Cavendish. Lord Anson, in the course of his voyage around the world, lost more than four-fifths of his men; and it is mentioned by Sir Richard Hawkins, that within his own naval experience, he had known more than ten thousand men perishing by the scurvy. Prior to the year 1796, more sailors, it is believed, fell victims to this terrific scourge, than to the united consequences of naval warfare and the various accidents incidental to a maritime life. These results, compared with the medical statistics of the Potomac's circumnavigation of the globe, we deem alone of sufficient importance in their deductions, to reward us for our present labor.